D1230980

HARDGAINERS'

BODYBUILDING HANDBOOK

Text ©2005 Hugo Rivera and Photographs ©2005 The Hatherleigh Company, Ltd.

No part of this book may be reproduced, stored in a retrieval system, or transmitted, in any form or by any means, electronic or otherwise, without written permission from the Publisher.

A GetFitNow.com Book
Published by Hatherleigh Press
5-22 46th Avenue, Suite 200
Long Island City, NY 11101
www.hatherleighpress.com

Library of Congress Cataloging-in-Publication Data

Rivera, Hugo A., 1974–
  Hardgainers' bodybuilding handbook: powerful secrets for gaining
muscle weight fast / by Hugo Rivera.
      p. cm.
  ISBN 1-57826-186-4
  1. Bodybuilding. 2. Exercise. 3. Muscle strength. I. Title.
  GV546.5.R58 2004
  613.7'13—dc22
                            2004021942

Disclaimer
All forms of exercise pose some inherent risks. The information in this book is meant to supplement, not replace, proper exercise training. Before practicing the exercises in this book, be sure that your equipment is well-maintained. Do not take risks beyond your level of experience, training, and fitness. The exercise and dietary programs in this book are not intended as a substitute for any exercise routine or treatment or dietary regimen that may have been prescribed by your doctor. As with all exercise and dietary programs, you should get your doctor's approval before beginning. The author, editors, and publisher advise readers to take full responsibility for their safety and know their limits.

GETFITNOW.COM BOOKS are available for bulk purchase, special promotions, and premiums. For information on reselling and special purchase opportunities, please call us at 1-800-528-2550 and ask the the Special Sales Manager.

Special thanks to Andre Hudson and Chris Lind.

Interior design by Deborah Miller
Cover design by Phil Mondestin and Deborah Miller

10 9 8 7 6 5 4 3 2 1
Printed in Canada

HARDGAINERS'

BODYBUILDING HANDBOOK

Hugo Rivera, BSCE, CFT, SPN

A GetFitNow.com Book

New York • London

DEDICATION

This book is dedicated to my beautiful wife Lina who always loves and supports me unconditionally throughout any project, to my son Chad who is my pride and joy and my biggest fan, to my parents and grandparents for always believing in me and who always ensured that I would get the best education possible as I was growing up, to my brother Raul whose computer knowledge made it possible for me to go online, to my in-laws who are always there to help me and provide me with support in time of need, to William Kemp for being such an awesome mentor and friend, to Chris Lind for all his awesome website assistance and friendship, to Tim and Brandie Gardner for always standing behind me on my fitness endeavors and for their friendship, and finally to God for giving me the talent to put this work together.

Hugo A. Rivera

Special thanks go out to:

Tim and Brandie Gardner for without your help, I would not be at the level of development that I am today. Also, I can't express my appreciation enough for allowing me to use your state-of-the-art facilities to perform the photo shoot of the exercises for this book. From the bottom of my heart, thank you so much for your expertise and great friendship!

Andre Hudson for being such an inspirational success story, an awesome trainer and a great friend. Also, many thanks to you and your family for making time to be part of the book's photo shoot. Can never thank you enough for your support.

Chris Lind for revamping my site, for your continued support, and also for all of the help in ensuring that the photo shoot would go so smoothly. Could not have done it without you!

Deborah Miller for sharing your expertise and talents with me, and thus, ensuring a most productive session. Look forward to working with you again in the future; we had a blast.

Peter Peck for being the most talented and passionate photographer I've ever met. It's truly an honor to work with someone of your caliber. As you know, I wish you the utmost success in all of your endeavors and thank you infinitely for all of the perfectionism and passion that you bring along with you when you do your work. It's truly inspiring to see you in action.

Laree and Dave Draper for always providing me with inspiration and for giving me my first endorsement in the industry back when IronOnline got started. Look forward to visiting you guys at your hometown in California this year.

Todd Mendelsohn who has also influenced my training tactics and who has played a key role as well on my development. When I think of training torture, I think about you. Always wishing you the best to you and your family.

Gene DellaSala, owner of audioholics.com, for undergoing rigorous testing of many of the training tactics that I use today back in the time when we were experimenting with different protocols. You have been one of the best training partners I've ever had and also an awesome friend.

The people at Prolab Inc. for giving me the opportunity to get more involved in the fitness industry and for putting out such awesome high quality products at a great price. Can't thank you guys enough.

To Andrea Au and Alyssa Smith for without your hard work and level of involvement in this project, this book would not be nearly the work it has become. I could not imagine working with better editors. Thank you so much for all of the long hours dedicated to this work!

To Andrew Flach and Kevin Moran for giving me the opportunity to spread the word of fitness to millions of people out there. I look forward to working with you guys in many projects to come.

Last but not least, to all of my fans out there, for without you, there would not be an audience to share my information with.

PRECAUTIONS

READ THIS SECTION THOROUGHLY BEFORE GOING ANY FURTHER!

- Always consult a physician before starting any weight gain or fat reduction training/nutrition program.

- A basic metabolic test, thyroid, lipid, and testosterone panel is recommended prior to starting this program to detect anything that could prevent getting the most out of your efforts. Consult your doctor regarding these tests.

- If you are unfamiliar with any of the exercises, consult an experienced trainer to instruct you on their proper form and execution. Improper form frequently leads to injury.

- The instructions and advice presented herein are not intended as a substitute for medical or other personal professional counseling.

- HR Fitness Inc., the editors, and authors disclaim any liability or loss in connection with the use of this system, its programs, and advice herein.

TABLE OF CONTENTS

CHAPTER 1:	The Science Behind Muscle Growth for the Hardgainer	1
CHAPTER 2:	Mass Building Training Tactics	7
CHAPTER 3:	Exercise Plan	17
CHAPTER 4:	Mass Building Nutrition	35
CHAPTER 5:	Supplementation for Maximum Growth	47
CHAPTER 6:	Rest and Recovery	65
CHAPTER 7:	Chest Exercises	73
CHAPTER 8:	Back Exercises	93
CHAPTER 9:	Shoulder Exercises	115
CHAPTER 10:	Biceps Exercises	135
CHAPTER 11:	Triceps Exercises	159
CHAPTER 12:	Quadriceps Exercises	175
CHAPTER 13:	Hamstring Exercises	193
CHAPTER 14:	Calf Exercises	217
CHAPTER 15:	Abdominal Exercises	235
CONCLUSION		255
APPENDIX A:	Meal Plan Schedule and Food Group Tables	257
APPENDIX B:	Food Journal and Diet Samples	262
APPENDIX C:	Break-In Routine	266
APPENDIX D:	Further Information about Creatine	272
APPENDIX E:	Glossary of Terms	274
APPENDIX F:	Websites and References	280
ABOUT THE AUTHOR		285

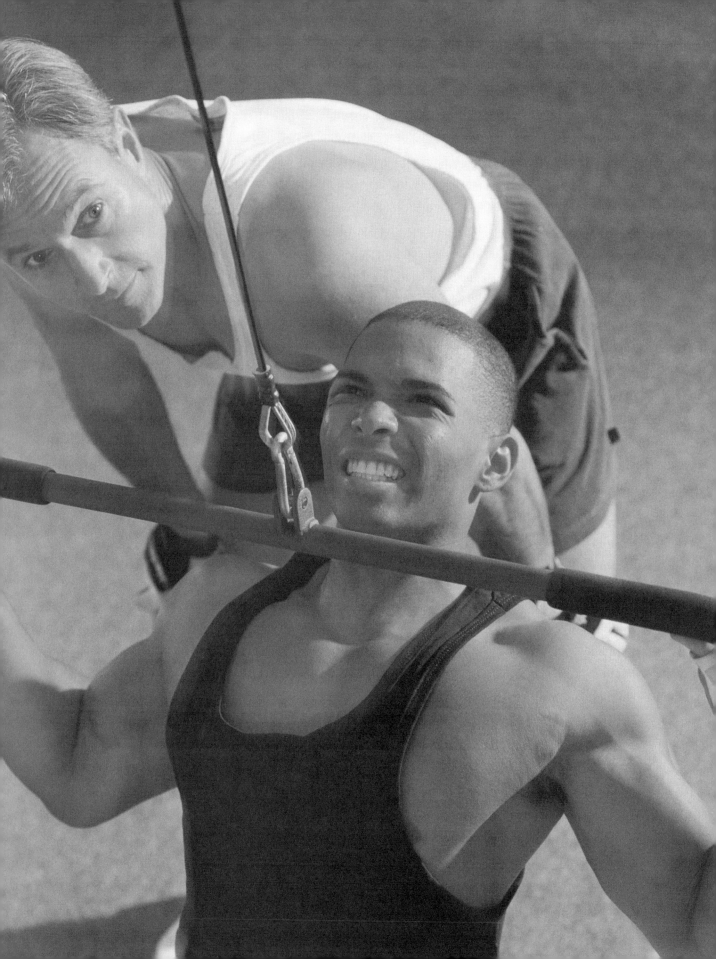

CHAPTER 1

The Science Behind Muscle Growth for the Hardgainer

If you are reading this book, you consider yourself a hardgainer. Maybe you were told by an "expert" at the gym that you do not have the genetics required to gain muscle, just as I was 15 years ago, or maybe you read about your body type in a muscle publication. Regardless of how you reached this conclusion, in this book I will cover what a hardgainer is and how to break the curse that prevents you from adding slabs of muscle to your frame. I can guarantee you that after reading this book you will be empowered with all the knowledge necessary for adding pounds of pure beef to your frame. How successful you ultimately become will rest in your determination to follow the plan until your goals are met.

Without much further ado, let's start by discussing what a hardgainer really is.

The Definition of a Hardgainer

Let me give you the popular definition and then my definition. The popular definition of a hardgainer is simply someone who works out hard with weights but has a difficult time putting on muscle. Six weeks of working out can go by with no significant changes in muscle size and only perhaps a bit of an increase in muscle tone. According to this broad definition, everyone is a hardgainer because putting on muscle is not an easy endeavor. The easiest period to gain muscle is during puberty. After that, gaining muscle becomes progressively harder as we age due to the fact that hormonal production starts declining between the ages of 25 and 30.

HARDGAINERS

My definition of a hardgainer is someone naturally skinny, who can eat practically anything and always seems to remain at the same body weight. Dr. William H. Sheldon referred to this bodytype as an ectomorph somatotype when he came up with his theory sometime in the 1940s. Sheldon's theory divides human bodies into three main somatotypes: the ectomorph, the endomorph, and the mesomorph. In a nutshell, the ectomorph is the naturally skinny person who has trouble gaining weight, whether in the form of muscle or fat. The endomorph, on the other hand, has the opposite problem, and it is too easy for a person with this body type to gain weight. While endomorphs are easy muscle gainers, provided they diet and train correctly, they are cursed with a slow metabolism, making it imperative that their diet be strict year round if they wish to have any abdominal definition. The final bodytype, the mesomorph, is the naturally muscular person, also favored with a higher metabolism than the endomorph. Mesomorphs make excellent bodybuilders and for them, gains in muscle and reduction in body fat come rather easily provided they maintain a great training and nutrition program. Life is not fair.

This book will concentrate on the ectomorph somatotype. While some people, especially endomorphs, consider the ectomorph's fast metabolism a blessing, for the ectomorph who wants to become a bodybuilder it is nothing short of a curse. I am not implying that the hardgainer is doomed to stay looking the same way forever; that, in fact, is the reason for the existence of this book. You can break away from your current physique and place yourself on the fast track to muscle gains. Will it be easy? No, but it is possible for you to add muscle mass. Fasten your seat belts and get ready for the ride of your life! By the time we are done you may not recognize the person looking back at you in the mirror.

The Importance of Goal Setting

In order to achieve the fastest results, you need measurable goals set every 12 weeks. Have you noticed people that go to the gym day in and day out and still look the same year after year? Typically, if you ask these people about their goals they either give you a blank stare or just tell you "I'm here to get in shape." I respect them for showing up to the gym as that alone is a feat by itself. But if you want to go somewhere you need to know where you are headed.

Imagine a boat in the middle of the ocean without a captain. Its course is blindly determined by the waves and the wind. If this boat ever gets somewhere it will be by random chance. Now, imagine for a moment the same boat with a cunning and determined captain. He sets a course on his map that will take him from point A to point B in the most expeditious manner. Needless to say, the captain will get to where he wants to go as fast as possible because he has a defined destination and also a plan to get there. He may encounter difficulties that may get him slightly off track, but because he has a mapped destination he can get himself back on track.

Bodybuilding is no different than navigating a boat. It is hard work and definitely not easy all the time. It requires having a final destination in mind and a plan that will allow you to get there. In order to achieve success in your program, your goals should be clearly defined. Otherwise, just like that lost ship, if you get anywhere it will be by chance.

I would like you to take out a small piece of paper right now and write down two things. The first will be your long-term goals. Be specific! Write the measurements that you will have (18-inch arms, 50-inch chest, 30-inch waist, 26-inch quads, 18-inch calves, etc.), your desired weight, and body fat percentage. Again, be specific! Don't limit yourself to what you think you can achieve; write down what you want. However, be realistic also. If you are 5'5" like myself you won't be able to have 25 inch arms or 35 inch quads. Only a bodybuilder that is 6'5", and possibly with chemical aid (e.g. steroids), can achieve that.

If you have moved on to this paragraph, you have written your long-term goals. The challenge lies in working towards those goals when they seem so far away. Well, every long trip starts with the first step. Write down your short-term goals. For the hardgainer, your short-term goals should be analyzed every 12 weeks. Short-term goals are going to be smaller than long-term goals, but they should still be as specific as possible. By identifying smaller short-term goals, you set the milestones to achieve your long-term goals. Whatever your goal, be positive and have no doubt in your mind that you can achieve it. This is crucial! So go ahead, right now, and write down your short-term goals. Do it in the following format:

For the next _____ (12 weeks) I will:
Gain _____ pounds of muscle
Weigh _____ pounds
Keep fat the same as muscle increases.

Have measurements of:

Chest/Back _____
Arms (right) _____
(left) _____
Waist _____
Thighs (right) _____
(left) _____
Calves (right) _____
(left) _____

Once you have all your goals written down, write down what ACTIONS you will take in the next 12 weeks to get there. For instance:

Action Plan:
- I will eat 3 balanced meals a day with three protein snacks.
- I will perform four weight-training sessions per week.
- I will perform two cardiovascular sessions per week.
- I will get 8 hours of sleep (7 minimum) every day.
- I will drink twelve to fifteen eight-ounce glasses of water a day.

If you want to, take pictures of how you currently look (be sure to also document current measurements, body weight, body fat, etc.). This is a great way to stay motivated, for when you look at pictures of yourself from your starting point, and then at pictures of yourself a year later, you will see a huge difference!

I also encourage making bi-weekly progress reports. Your reports allow you to accurately track the progress you make. Checking your progress on a bi-weekly basis will encourage you to work harder to reach your goals. If you find that you are not gaining weight, these reports let you
troubleshoot your diet and fix any issue before the 12-week program is complete. I personally take pictures, body fat readings, and measurements every couple of weeks when on a mass gaining phase (what this book is all about). However, if I am dieting for a contest, I take weekly readings and pictures so that if something stops working, I can fix the problem as soon as possible. Later in the book, I will show you how to troubleshoot your diet and nutrition in case that you do not make progress.

Now that we have discussed your goals and how to track them, and have a written plan for the future, it is time to get to the actions that will take you there. If you follow your action plan religiously but you miss your goals by a bit, DON'T GET DISCOURAGED! You should see progress anyway and this is what we are shooting for (and here is where pictures really pay off—it may be a good idea to purchase a digital camera). Constant progress is what will get you to the goals you want to achieve.

If you missed your mark because you did not follow your action plan to the letter, don't punish yourself for it. Set your new goals and be more determined in following your action plan to get you there the next time.

Muscle Growth Formula for Success

Now that we have discussed the importance of setting goals, we need to talk about the factors that will impact your ability to reach them. These factors are described by the muscle growth formula for success. If any of the factors in this formula are not optimized, then it will take longer for you to reach your goals. It's like having an engine that is not operating at peak efficiency because it needs an oil change.

Muscle Growth Success = Determination x (Nutrition + Training + Rest)

A value of 1 is given to a component if it is followed completely. A value of 0 is given to any component that is not followed or followed halfway. If every single component is followed, the result is a maximum muscle growth success value of 3. A 3 is a person that will get the fastest results possible from this program. If the person stops following one of the components, they will get a smaller muscle growth success value and less than optimal results. Note that if you don't have any determination you get a muscle growth success value of 0. If you are not determined to do something, the first obstacle that comes your way will get you off track for good.

Life is not perfect and it certainly does not adjust itself so that we can have an easy time achieving our personal goals. You will need to be determined, set a plan, and follow through with it no matter what happens. Obstacles will come. Once they do, it is your determination to achieve your goal that will give you the motivation to face the obstacle, determine a plan of action, and push forward. There is nothing that can stop you from achieving something if you are determined enough to do it. On the other hand, if you are not determined, the slightest setback will make you quit your program and have no gains as a result.

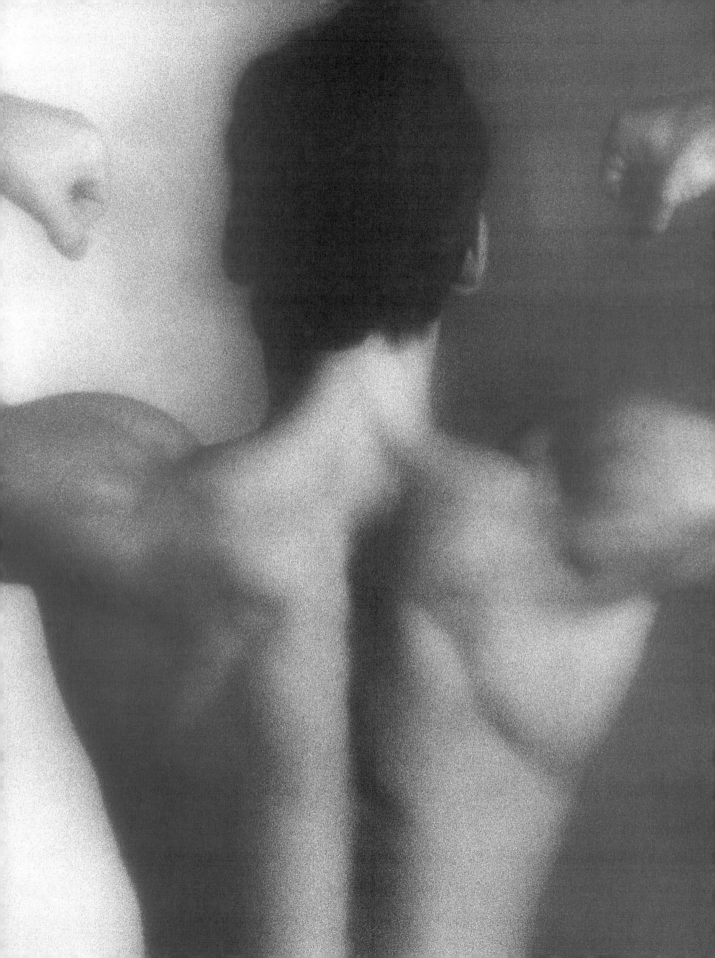

CHAPTER 2
Mass Building Training Tactics

If you're looking to spark muscle growth, eventually you're going to have to learn the basics of bodybuilding training. This chapter is designed to give you an overview of these tenets, and, accompanied by proper nutrition and a training plan, that will place you on the road to success.

Mass Building Training Principles

Sessions should be short: 60 minutes maximum. The maximum amount of time a weight training session should last is 60 minutes. After 60 minutes, levels of muscle-building hormones like testosterone begin to drop. The fuel your muscles use to contract, stored carbohydrates in your liver and muscle cells known as glycogen, is depleted as well after 60 minutes. If you weight train more than 60 minutes you will waste your time since your body no longer has the hormones or the fuel necessary to produce muscle growth. Training past 60 minutes leads to impaired recovery and possibly overtraining, a condition where your body does not recover from its weight training sessions. Overtraining generally results in loss of strength and muscle mass.

The rest between sets should be kept to a minimum; 90 seconds or less. Keeping your rest time between exercises low not only allows you to perform a large amount of work within the 60-minute weight training window, but also has health benefits. It helps improve your cardiovascular system, and most importantly, maximizes the output of growth hormone; a powerful fat burning/muscle building hormone. This rest interval also promotes a muscle voluminizing effect on the cellular level, sending water inside the muscle cells and makes the muscles look more firm and toned. This is completely unlike water retention outside of the muscle cells, which makes bodybuilders look puffy and fat.

Weight training exercise should not be performed for more than two days in a row. This is essential for hardgainers. While most endomorphs can recover from a six-day per week training split, most hardgainers have difficulty recovering from more than four sessions per week. Their nervous systems become very taxed after two days of high intensity weight training, so continuing to train for more than two days leads to depressing the nervous system. This prevents the body from recruiting all the muscle fibers they ordinarily could while performing a lift. In addition, with a constantly depressed nervous system, strength gains not only become impossible to come by, but also impossible to keep. As a result you could see your strength diminishing.

Sets of each exercise should consist of a range of 6–15 repetitions. The most important reason for this is that within this range the growth hormone output is maximized. This is a good thing since this hormone does exactly what we are looking for—increasing muscle and decreasing body fat. In addition, because you are performing so many repetitions, you get a great pump (blood rushing into the muscle). This provides nutrients to nourish muscle cells and helps them recover and rebuild faster. Finally, performing 6–15 repetitions reduces the possibility of injury dramatically since you will need to use a weight that you can control in order to perform the number of reps. (Note: This rule does not apply to the calves and abdominals as these muscles usually respond better to higher repetition ranges, in the order of 13–15 reps).

Training must be progressive. Progression means the exercise should get increasingly more difficult from session to session. Another repetition might be added, or more weight could be placed on the lift if 15 repetitions have been reached. However, it is important to understand that you will not be able to increase the weight or the number of repetitions every session. Progression comes in many forms, like performing more work within the 60-minute period. The overarching goal of a training routine is to ensure progress over a period of time to bring about continuous improvements in muscle mass and definition.

Training must be varied. This principle is vital to ensure continuous gains in strength and muscle tone, as well as a more basic aim of preventing boredom. Variation does not mean changing all of the exercises in your program. You could use different techniques to stimulate the muscle, change repetition and set parameters, change the rest between sets, or even something as simple as changing the width of your grip placement on the bar to help isolate specific muscles. In this program you will alternate between 3-week periods of high volume work and 3-week periods of higher intensity (heavier weights) work. In this manner, the body is stressed in a manner that allows for its maximum growth stimulus. If you were to perform the same lifting routine day in and day out, the result would be stagnation, because a routine only works for as long as it takes the body to adapt to it.

The form in which you perform an exercise should be impeccable. By letting the ego take control, many lifters concentrate on increasing the weight without regard to exercise form. Not only can this practice seriously injure the muscles being trained, sometimes even requiring surgery, but also it prevents proper stimulation of the muscles being trained. When form is less than perfect, other muscle groups come in and assist in the exercise and take away some of the force from the muscle supposedly being targeted. This practice slows down growth and could get you seriously injured, so please pay close attention to your exercise form.

Aerobic exercise and outside activities should be minimized. While I am not anti-aerobics by any means, and actually love to walk, ride my bike, and do other activities to keep my cardiovascular system in shape, this is a tricky point with the hardgainer. In order for the hardgainer to maximize results in muscle mass, aerobic activity and other activities such as high activity sports (basketball, soccer, and others,) need to be minimized. The reason for this goes right back to nervous system recovery and the hardgainer's super fast metabolism. By erforming too many caloric burning activities, you make it harder on yourself to gain muscle. You will need more caloric than what is recommended in this book in order to cover your energy needs and also those required by muscle growth. In this book, we suggest limiting cardiovascular activity to a couple of times per week from 15 minutes to no more than 25.

Training must consist primarily of free weight basic exercises. Only free weight basic exercises can provide the fast results you are looking for because they recruit the most muscle into the lifts. The body is designed to be in a three dimensional universe, and whenever you use a machine it limits your body to two-dimensions and consequently limits the muscle fibers that can train. However, not all machines are bad, and some definitely have a place in our weight-training program. These few allow us to isolate a muscle in a way that no free weights could allow. The program here will be based on barbell, dumbbell, and exercises where the body moves through space, such as the dip, the pull-up, and the squat. In the sections below, we will detail which exercises are the best for muscle gains and the reasons behind it.

The Best Exercises for Mass Gains

Which exercises are the best ones for mass gains? I am asked this question on an almost daily basis.

There are a variety of exercises that you can select to sculpt the body of your dreams. Results in bodybuilding are generally measured in body composition changes: increased muscle mass or tone, depending on the goal, along with decreases in body fat. The speed at which such changes are acquired depends on the training protocol used, the nutrition plan followed, and the amount of rest (good night's sleep) that the trainee gets.

In order for a training protocol to work at peak efficiency, not only must it work over a period or cycle but it also must include exercises that give you the most stimulation in the minimum amount of time.

Different exercises provide different levels of stimulation. Exercises like the leg extensions, while excellent for sculpting the lower part of the quadriceps, produce less of a stimulating effect than an exercise like the squat. The efficiency of an exercise, then, really depends on the exercise's ability to involve the maximum amount of muscle fibers and on its ability to provide a neuromuscular stimulation (NMS).

Neuromuscular stimulation is extremely important as it is the nervous system that sends the signal to the brain requesting the start of the muscle growth process. Having said that, how do we determine the stimulation factor of each exercise?

The NMS Classes

The rating of the NMS exercises is based in a ranking system. In our exercise rating system composed of four classes, a class 1 exercise yields the lowest NMS (this class is composed of variable resistance machine type of exercises) while a class 4 exercise yields the highest NMS and is therefore the hardest but most stimulating one. In each class we may also have subclasses such as class 1a and class 1b. A class 1a exercise will yield less NMS than a class 1b.

Class 1a

Class 1a exercises are composed of isolation (one joint) exercises performed in variable resistance machines (such as Nautilus) where the whole movement of the exercise is controlled. These type of exercises provide the least amount of stimulation as stabilizer muscles are not involved and the machine takes care of the stabilization process. An example of such an exercise would be the machine curl.

Class 1b

Class 1b exercises are compound (multi-joint) movements performed in a variable resistance machine. An example of such movement would be the incline bench press performed in a Hammer Strength machine. Since the movement is a compound one, more muscles are involved and therefore the neuromuscular stimulation is higher than that offered by a machine curl. However, the fact that the machine takes care of stabilization issue limits the growth offered by the exercise.

Class 2a

Class 2a exercises are composed of isolation (one joint) exercises performed with non-variable-resistance machines. An example of such exercise would be the leg extension exercise as seen on benches sold for home gyms (a leg extensions attachment). These attachments lack the pulleys and cams that would make the exercise a variable resistance exercise. Therefore, the muscles need to get more involved in the movement, something that provides better stimulation.

Class 2b

Class 2b exercises are basic (multi-joint) exercises performed with non-variable resistance machines.

An example would be the bench press unit attached to the Universal machines, or a leg press machine that contains no pulleys or cams. Without pulleys or cams to make the exercise easier as you lift the weight, the NMS is higher.

Class 3a

Class 3a exercises are isolation (one joint) exercises performed with free weights. One example could be a concentration curl performed with a dumbbell. It is still not clear whether a multi-joint exercise performed on a machine offers the same amount or better NMS than the one offered by a free weight isolation exercise. However, for the purposes of this discussion, we will assume that the free weight isolation exercise provides more stimulation as stabilizer muscles come into play (especially if you do the exercise standing up).

Class 3b

Class 3b exercises are multi-jointed basic exercises performed with barbell free weights.

Class 3c

Class 3c exercises are multi-jointed basic exercises performed with dumbbell free weights. The barbell exercises provide less NMS as the movement is more restrained as opposed to dumbbells where the weights can go in all types of directions unless all of your stabilizer muscles jump in and constrain the movement. Because of this, dumbbells provide the highest NMS in this category.

Class 4

Finally, class 4 exercises, the king of exercises, are free weight exercises in which your body moves through space. In other words, this could be any exercise where your torso is moving. This could be squats, deadlifts, pull-ups, close grip chins, push-ups, lunges, or dips, all which provide the most stimulation possible and therefore, the fastest results. To prove this simply, have you ever noticed how many people do great amounts of weights in a pulldown machine but have trouble doing pull-ups?

In order for you to perform these types of free space exercises, you need to be capable of not only carrying the added resistance but also of involving your body weight. Many muscles are called into play to perform this feat. By performing dips, chinups, squats, and deadlifts, you hit every single muscle in your body! These exercises not only give you fast results, but they create functional strength; strength that can be used for your daily activities.

If you are great at performing pull-ups and you go to perform a pull-down you'll see how easy the task of performing a pull-down is. As a matter of fact, depending on your pull-up strength, you might be able to lift the whole stack in most pulldown machines. However, the reverse is not true. While you may be very good at performing pulldowns, you may not be able to perform many pull-ups as the strength gained in the pulldown exercise is not as transferable as the one gained in a pull-up. Again, the reason for this phenomenon is NMS.

Workout Periodization: The Hardgainer's Secret Weapon

Your next weapon in the fight to increase muscle mass is to periodize your workouts. Periodization is nothing more than cycling your workout parameters of sets, repetitions, rest in between sets, and the exercises themselves. Extremely successful bodybuilders learn to do this almost instinctively. Arnold Schwarzenegger was known for continually changing his workouts on almost a daily basis. In addition, he had a full year plan that cycled his intensity levels, all designed to peak him for his Mr. Olympia contest once a year.

Having said this, it is not enough to change a thing or two in your workouts in order to continually grow. Instead, by changing your workout parameters in an orderly and logical manner you can maximize results in the gym and avoid stagnation.

There are two ways the muscle can be stimulated: volume training and strength training.

VOLUME TRAINING

Volume is the number of sets times the number of repetitions per set. If you perform a routine for chest that consists of 10 sets of 10 reps of an incline barbell press, then your total volume was 100 reps. A typical training of this type calls for 8-12 sets per body part (if trained once per week) and 8-20 repetitions per set. The maximum suggested rest time is 1 minute per set, and thus the use of supersets is valuable in this training phase. How does volume training work? An increase in workout volume yields the following adaptations:

- The growth hormone output increases because of the short rest interval between sets, and the high volume.
- Hypertrophy (muscle growth) occurs when the body increases the levels of creatine phosphate (CP), water, and carbohydrates inside the muscle cell. This muscle voluminization happens as a result of short rest intervals and cumulative fatigue caused by the total number of sets. You see, short rest intervals do not allow the full replenishment of the energy system that is responsible for allowing muscle contractions to occur; namely adenosine tri-phosphate (ATP) and creatine phosphate (CP). Because of this, the body becomes more efficient at increasing its energy transport capability. It does this through an increase in creatine phosphate and glycogen (stored carbohydrates) levels inside the muscle cell. As a result, the muscle cell gets bigger and the protein synthesis mechanisms get activated, creating muscle hypertrophy as a result.
- The body's recuperation capabilities are increased due to the stress imposed by the multiplying work coupled with short rest intervals.

Unfortunately, even though volume training works this well, we can't train like this all the time. It requires a high volume of work, which, if kept up for too long, will eventually result in overtraining and injury. In addition the body adjusts to anything that remains constant, and thus we need to eventually change to a cycle of strength training.

STRENGTH TRAINING

In a strength training phase, the focus is on intensity, or the amount of weight used in a lift. A typical phase will consist of 8-10 sets per body part and 8-4 repetitions per set. Modified compound supersets are usually used in order to save time while resting 3 minutes or more for a particular lift.

- The testosterone levels increase in response to the longer rest period between sets, and stress from the heavier weights.
- Hypertrophy (muscle growth) occurs when the body increases the actual diameter of the muscle fiber through increased protein synthesis. Spoken simply, the actual protein content of the cell increases, as does the thickness of the muscle filaments. In this phase, strength gains come first and muscle growth later.
- Your body's increased recuperation abilities (gained from the previous phase and its regime of lowered volume) are used to increase strength and build more muscle mass. Your body will adapt to prepare itself for another stressful strength-gaining period.

Without a strength training phase, muscle would grow but never as a result of actual fiber growth—only as a result of intracellular fluids such as CP, glycogen, water, etc. In addition, your muscle would never be as strong as it looks due to the fact that strength training phases are required in order to teach the nervous system to recruit the fast twitch (white) fibers which are responsible for massive strength. Therefore, it is of utmost importance that you incorporate strength-training phases in your periodization plan for muscle growth.

ACTIVE RECOVERY TRAINING

There is a third type of training that is called active recovery training. While not a phase that stimulates muscle growth, unless you are an absolute beginner, this phase is a necessary part of training. The active recovery phase has three main functions:

- First, according to leading strength expert Tudor Bompa, Ph.D., "you are trying to adapt the anatomy of the body to the upcoming training so that you can create, or produce an injury free environment". Essentially, this step is to ensure your tendons and ligaments are strong enough to support the stressful periods that will follow.
- Second, this phase is a great time to address any strength imbalance that your body might have. Dumbbells, as the most flexible piece of exercise equipment, are used during this phase.
- Finally, this phase also acts as a time for the body to re-charge its energy stores and allow for complete physical and mental recuperation.

Typically, this phase is a week-long session that is used directly after 6 weeks of intense training.

How Fast Should You Lift the Weight?

Slow lifting is only helpful for the beginners who have never lifted before. If you are a beginner, your movements should be slow and deliberate in order to allow your nervous system to learn how to coordinate lifting the weight correctly. In addition, slow lifting prevents the trainee from using bad exercise form.

As you become more advanced, science and my own experience tell you to lift the weight as fast as possible throughout the concentric movement (the portion of the movement when the muscle contracts) without sacrificing form and without involving flawed momentum (jerking and bouncing of the weights). The eccentric portion (the portion where the muscle lengthens) should be performed slowly and deliberately.

Why a fast concentric movement? You create more force by trying to lift fast. In order to create that force, more muscle fibers are activated to move the weight at a faster speed. By ensuring that you are not using momentum to move the weight, all of the force is created by your muscles and stimulates them to grow. While super slow lifting hurts, it is not the best way to stimulate muscle growth since all it does is accumulate lactic acid in your muscles and fatigue them before they reach real failure. Science tells us that Force = Mass (in this case the weight you are lifting) x Acceleration (the increasing speed at which you lift the weight). Therefore, as long as momentum is not included in the equation, and the weight is lifted fast but with total control, this is the best way to lift weights. Since you won't be jerking the weights, the risk of getting injured is not any bigger than the risk of getting injured lifting super slowly. However, if you are lifting a weight that only allows you to do 5 repetitions, it will appear as if you are lifting the weight slowly even though you are lifting it as fast as possible. The fact that the heavier the weight, the slower you will be able to move it, even if you are trying to accelerate it as fast as you can.

How To Breathe While Performing The Exercise

The correct way to breathe while performing an exercise is to exhale (breathe out) during the concentric portion of the movement and to inhale (breathe in) when you are lowering the weight during the eccentric portion. For example, if you are doing a bench press, you breathe in while you lower the weight and breathe out when you start moving the weight away from your chest.

Missing Workouts

Missing workouts is unacceptable. There are 24 hours in a day and there is always a way to work out provided you have determination. Missing workouts jeopardizes your growth and destroys a bodybuilder's mindset. However, if for some reason you are not able to train (because all of the gyms in the world are closed on that day, and you have no gym or dumbbells at home and don't know anyone with one) then make up the missed session the next day. However, it is still essential you do not train more than 2 days in a row. Since you are working out 4 days per week, if you miss a training session, all you have to do is move the whole program forward by a day, which will have you doing your last session of the week on a Saturday. For instance, let's say that Monday was super hectic at the office and by the time you came out the gym was closed. Then in this case, your workout schedule will be Tuesday, Wednesday, Friday, and Saturday. When Monday comes around, then you can start over as normal. If Tuesday is missed, then perform the routine on Wednesday, rest Thursday, and workout on Friday and Saturday. When Monday rolls around you are back on track again.

Aerobic Training

Aerobic training such as walking or running on a stationary bike is a good way to keep the cardio-vascular system running and to minimize fat gains while gaining mass as long as it is not overdone.

The fat burning zone is the exercise level at which you are doing enough work to burn fat. Your pulse (how fast your heart is beating per minute) determines this zone. The fat burning zone formula is the following:

Fat burning zone=220-(your age) x (.75)

The result of your formula will give you an approximate value of how fast your heart should be beating per minute. For example, a 20-year-old would need to reach a pulse in the neighborhood of 150 beats per minute in order to be in the fat burning zone. It is important to remember that

this is not an absolute figure, so as long as you are plus or minus 10 beats from the number that the formula provides, you will be burning fat.

For bodybuilders in contest training or fitness enthusiasts who are just trying to lose weight, typically I recommend that they perform cardio either in the morning on an empty stomach or after the workout. Both of these times the body is depleted of glycogen, thus facilitating fat loss. However, for the hardgainer the best way to go is any time of the day, to prevent catabolism (muscle loss). Hardgainers must be very careful with putting out too much effort so please do not go above the fat burning zone.

Aerobic Exercise Recommendations

I recommend a couple of sessions a week for 20-25 minutes as this should suffice for the hardgainer. The goal is again to just keep the cardiovascular system healthy and to keep fat gains at bay. I suggest performing your cardio on Wednesdays and Saturdays on the afternoons when you typically do your weights on weight training days or any other convenient time.

Good forms of aerobic exercise are: stationary bike, fast walking (also can be done on a treadmill), stairstepper, fitness rider, rowing machine, or any other form of cardiovascular activity that would raise your heartbeat to the fat burning zone. If you feel that you are an extreme hardgainer with a super fast metabolism just stick to walking, as this is the aerobic activity that burns the fewest of calories.

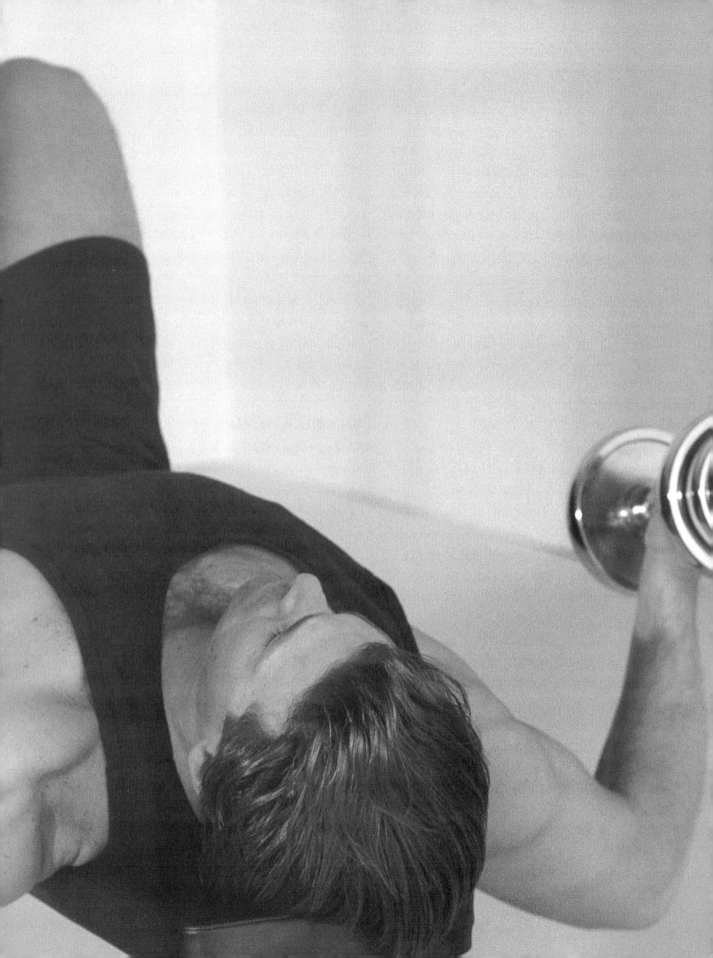

CHAPTER 3

Exercise Plan

Hardgainer's Training Model

Creating a periodization model that will maximize the muscle producing capabilities of each training model is by far the most difficult part of preparing your plan.

Since our main goal is muscle growth, the dominant tactic in the periodization model will be volume training. Starting with an active recovery phase followed by 6 weeks of volume training, called the hypertrophy phase, we will follow this with a 1 week active recovery phase, and 6 more weeks of the hypertrophy phase. Next is another active recovery phase followed by 3 weeks of a hybrid phase, where both Volume Training and Strength Training will be used. The cycle is finished with a 3-week pure Strength Training phase. The chart below shows you how your periodization model will look:

HARDGAINER'S PERIODIZATION MODEL	
Type of Phase	**Phase Duration**
ACTIVE RECOVERY PHASE	1 WEEK
HYPERTROPHY PHASE (VOLUME TRAINING)	6 WEEKS
ACTIVE RECOVERY PHASE	1 WEEK
HYPERTROPHY PHASE (VOLUME TRAINING)	6 WEEKS
ACTIVE RECOVERY PHASE	1 WEEK
HYBRID PHASE (VOLUME/STRENGTH TRAINING)	3 WEEK
STRENGTH PHASE (STRENGTH TRAINING)	3 WEEK
START OVER	

After developing a periodization model that suits our purpose, it's just a matter of creating routines that use all of the theories discussed so far. Keep in mind that these routines were developed for people that have at least 5 months of training experience. If this is not the case, then please use the break-in routine presented below. Don't get frustrated! Even though you won't use the actual program, you will still make fantastic gains because your body is not used to weight training at all. Get ready to grow!

DAYS OF THE WEEK

You'll see that I have specified days of the week for each workout. I've found that this schedule works best for those of us dealing with a Monday through Friday workweek. However, if you need to alter the schedule, you should certainly feel free to do so. Just be sure to keep the workouts in sequence and don't work out more than 2 days in a row. Because these workouts are very intense, you need to give your muscles some time to rest and recover.

Hardgainer's Muscle Mass Accumulation Training Model

We have finally arrived at the presentation of the training model that incorporates all of the principles covered so far. While many other routines could be developed to follow the tenets, we went with the best routines available, routines that have been proven time and time again. If for some reason you cannot perform a prescribed exercise due to injury or unavailability of equipment, simply substitute a similar exercise that targets the same muscle group.

Active Recovery Phase #1

DURATION: 1 WEEK

Purpose: Allows for recovery of the body from previous training, priming it for the muscle-building phase.

Training Methodology: Fast-paced full body routine consisting largely of dumbbells to allow for maximum involvement of all muscles as well as to correct any strength imbalances in the body.

MONDAY/THURSDAY			FULL BODY ROUTINE	
EXERCISE	**PAGE NO.**	**REPS**	**SETS**	**REST**
SUPERSET # 1				
Incline Dumbbell Press	74	13-15	2	No Rest
Pull-down to Front	94	13-15	2	1 minute
SUPERSET # 2				
Dumbbell Bench Press	76	13-15	2	No Rest
One Arm Dumbbell Rows	96	13-15	2	1 minute
SUPERSET # 3				
Bent-over Lateral Raises	122	13-15	2	No Rest
Dumbbell Shoulder Press	116	13-15	2	1 minute
SUPERSET # 4				
Incline Dumbbell Curls	140	13-15	2	No Rest
Overhead Dumbbell Triceps Extensions	164	13-15	2	1 minute
SUPERSET # 5				
Squats	177	13-15	2	No Rest
Lying Leg Curls	204	13-15	2	1 minute
SUPERSET # 6				
Leg Extensions	182	13-15	2	No Rest
Standing Calf Raises	218	13-15	2	1 minute
SUPERSET #7				
Lying Leg Raises	240	13-15	2	No Rest
Crunches	238	13-15	2	1 minute

Hypertrophy Phase #1: Volume Training
WEEKS: 2–7
DURATION: 6 WEEKS

Purpose: Increase the body's muscle mass levels through an intra-cellular increase of energy substrates and water.

Training Methodology: For this phase, the 10 sets of 10 method and the 8 sets of 8 method were selected. Both methods have been proven to be fantastic at increasing muscle mass as muscles are systematically fatigued. For the 10 x 10 routine, a mass building exercise is chosen and a weight that you are able to use for 15 reps is selected. However, you will stop at 10 reps. If you keep the same weight for all ten sets, once fatigue sets in, you will find the sets more and more challenging. The 8 x 8 routine will be used in the same manner, except you will select a weight that you can use for 12-13 reps.

For both routines, one additional exercise is selected that serves as an active recovery exercise for the remaining upper body or lower body parts not trained directly that day.

MONDAY				CHEST/BACK/TRAPS
EXERCISE	**PAGE NO.**	**REPS**	**SETS**	**REST**
SUPERSET # 1				
Incline Barbell Press	78	10	10	No Rest
Pull-up To Front (wide grip)	98	10	10	1 minute
NOTES: If you cannot perform the wide grip pull-up, then have your partner help you up or use a weight assist machine. Otherwise, substitute wide grip pull-downs.				
SUPERSET # 2				
Chest Dips	80	15–20	2	No Rest
Close Grip Chins	100	15–20	2	1 minute
NOTES: This superset also indirectly works the biceps and the triceps.				
SUPERSET # 3				
Lateral Raises	128	15–20	2	No Rest
Upright Rows	120	15–20	2	1 minute

TUESDAY — HAMSTRINGS/CALVES/LOWER ABS

EXERCISE	PAGE NO.	REPS	SETS	REST
SUPERSET # 1 Lying Leg Curls	204	10	10	No Rest
Lying Leg Raises	240	10	10	1 minute
NOTES: For the lying leg raises, use the smallest dumbbell you can find and hold with your feet. If you are unable to use a weight, perform the exercise without it.				
Dumbbell Lunges (press with heel)	196	15–20	2	1 minute
Standing Calf Raises	218	15–20	8	30 seconds

THURSDAY — BICEPS/TRICEPS/DELTS

EXERCISE	PAGE NO.	REPS	SETS	REST
SUPERSET # 1 Incline Dumbbell Curls	140	8	8	No Rest
Lying Triceps Extensions	166	8	8	1 minute
Dumbbell Shoulder Press	116	8	8	1 minute
SUPERSET # 2 Neutral Grip Chin-Ups	136	15–20	2	No Rest
Close Grip Bench Press	160	15–20	2	1 minute
Bent-over Lateral Raises	122	15–20	2	No Rest

FRIDAY — QUADRICEPS/CALVES/UPPER ABS

EXERCISE	PAGE NO.	REPS	SETS	REST
SUPERSET # 1 Squats (medium stance)	177	10	10	No Rest
Crunches	238	10	10	1 minute
NOTES: In the crunches, use the smallest weight you can find and hold with your arms extended in front. If you are not strong enough to use a weight, perform without it.				
Squats (wide stance)	177	15–20	2	1 minute
NOTES: You may substitute wide stance leg presses if you have lower back problems. Same goes for the medium stance squats above.				
Calf Press	220	8	8	30 seconds

Active Recovery Phase #2

DURATION: 1 WEEK

Purpose: Allows for recovery of the body to prime it for the muscle-building phase.

Training Methodology: Fast-paced full body routine consisting largely of dumbbells to allow for maximum involvement of all muscles as well as to correct any strength imbalances in the body.

MONDAY/THURSDAY			FULL BODY ROUTINE	
EXERCISE	**PAGE NO.**	**REPS**	**SETS**	**REST**
SUPERSET # 1				
Incline Dumbbell Press	74	13–15	2	No Rest
Pull-down to Front	94	13–15	2	1 minute
SUPERSET # 2				
Dumbbell Bench Press	76	13–15	2	No Rest
One Arm Dumbbell Rows	96	13–15	2	1 minute
SUPERSET # 3				
Bent-over Lateral Raises	122	13–15	2	No Rest
Dumbbell Shoulder Press	116	13–15	2	1 minute
SUPERSET # 4				
Incline Dumbbell Curls	140	13–15	2	No Rest
Overhead Dumbbell Triceps Extensions	164	13–15	2	1 minute
SUPERSET # 5				
Squats	177	13–15	2	No Rest
Lying Leg Curls	204	13–15	2	1 minute
SUPERSET # 6				
Leg Extensions	182	13–15	2	No Rest
Standing Calf Raises	218	13–15	2	1 minute
SUPERSET #7				
Lying Leg Raises	240	13–15	2	No Rest
Crunches	238	13–15	2	1 minute

Hypertrophy Phase #2: Volume Training

WEEKS: 9–14
DURATION: 6 WEEKS

Purpose: Increase the body's muscle mass levels through an intra-cellular increase of energy substrates and water.

Training Methodology: The last Hypertrophy Phase concentrated on the 10 sets of 10 method and the 8 sets of 8 method, and one angle of attack. This phase attacks the muscle from different angles in order to activate many different muscle fibers. Like the other methods presented so far, this has been used instinctively by many bodybuilders, such as Arnold Schwarzenegger. This method is also very popular with Florida's bodybuilding guru Tim Gardner. The reason this multi-angular approach works is because the muscle is worked through all its ranges of motion; the midrange, stretched, and contracted ranges. When you train a muscle through its full range of motion, muscle fiber recruitment is maximized. To select a weight for your exercises, choose one that allows you to perform the exercise with good form for the required amount of reps. The last repetition should be challenging but not impossible.

MONDAY		CHEST/BACK/TRAPS/REAR DELTS		
EXERCISE	**PAGE NO.**	**REPS**	**SETS**	**REST**
SUPERSET # 1				
Incline Barbell Press	78	6-8	3	No Rest
Pull-up to Front (wide grip)	98	6-8	3	1 minute
NOTES: If you cannot perform the wide grip pull-up, then have your partner help you up or use a weight assist machine. Otherwise, substitute wide grip pull-downs.				
SUPERSET # 2				
Chest Dips	80	6-8	3	No Rest
Close Grip Chins	100	6-8	3	1 minute
NOTES: This superset indirectly works the biceps and the triceps as well.				
SUPERSET # 3				
Cable Incline Flies	82	10-12	3	No Rest
Low Pulley Rows	106	10-12	3	No Rest
Dumbbell Pullovers	84	10-12	2	1 minute
NOTES: The stretch portion of the low pulley rows should be emphasized as well. Note the last superset you perform will consist of only the first two exercises.				
SUPERSET # 4				
Stiff-Arm Pull-downs	108	15-20	2	No Rest
Bent Arm Bent-over Rows	124	15-20	2	No Rest
Upright Rows	120	15-20	2	No Rest

HARDGAINERS

TUESDAY				HAMSTRINGS/CALVES/ABS
EXERCISE	**PAGE NO.**	**REPS**	**SETS**	**REST**
SUPERSET # 1				
Hamstrings Leg Press	198	6-8	4	No Rest
Hanging Leg Raises	242	10-15	3	1 minute
NOTES: Note the last superset you perform will consist of only the first exercise.				
SUPERSET # 2				
Dumbbell Stiff-Legged Deadlifts	200	10-12	4	No Rest
Bicycle Crunches	244	15	3	1 minute
NOTES: Note that the last superset you perform will consist of only the first exercise.				
SUPERSET # 3				
Lying Leg Curls	204	10-12	4	No Rest
Crunches	238	10-15	3	30 seconds
NOTES: Note that the last superset you perform will consist of only the first exercise.				
SUPERSET # 4				
Donkey Calf Raises	222	10-15	4	No Rest
Standing Calf Raises	218	8	3	30 seconds
NOTES: If no donkey calf raises are available in your gym, calf raises using the leg press machine are acceptable. If you cannot superset these exercises due to gym set-up, perform each separately with 30 seconds of rest between sets.				

THURSDAY — BICEPS/TRICEPS/DELTS

EXERCISE	PAGE NO.	REPS	SETS	REST
SUPERSET # 1				
Close Grip Chins	100	6–8	3	No Rest
Close Grip Bench Press	160	6–8	3	1 minute
NOTES: For chin-ups, emphasize lifting your body using your biceps. If you cannot perform this exercise, have your partner assist or use a weight assist machine. Otherwise, perform close grip pull-downs. For the close grip bench presses, emphasize training your triceps.				
SUPERSET # 2				
Incline Dumbbell Curls	140	10–12	3	No Rest
Overhead Dumbbell Triceps Extensions	164	10–12	3	1 minute
SUPERSET # 3				
Concentration Curls	142	15–20	3	No Rest
Triceps Kickbacks	168	15–20	3	1 minute
SUPERSET # 4				
Seated Military Press	118	8	3	No Rest
Incline One Arm Laterals	126	10–12	3	No Rest
Lateral Raises	128	15–20	3	1 minute

FRIDAY — QUADRICEPS/CALVES/ABS

EXERCISE	PAGE NO.	REPS	SETS	REST
SUPERSET # 1				
Squats (medium stance)	177	6–8	4	No Rest
Hanging Leg Raises	242	10–15	3	1 minute
NOTES: If you suffer from low back problems, use the leg press machine with a medium stance instead of the medium stance squats and press with your toes to emphasize the quads. Note that the last superset you perform will only consist of the first exercise.				
SUPERSET # 2				
Sissy Squats	184	10–12	4	No Rest
Bicycle Crunches	244	15	3	1 minute
NOTES: Note that the last superset you perform will only consist of the first exercise.				
SUPERSET # 3				
Leg Extensions	182	15–20	4	No Rest
Crunches	238	10–15	3	1 minute
NOTES: Note that the last superset you perform will consist of only the first exercise.				
SUPERSET # 4				
Donkey Calf Raises	222	10–15	4	No Rest
Standing Calf Raises	218	8	4	30 seconds
NOTES: If no donkey calf raises are available in your gym, calf raises using the leg press machine may replace them. If you cannot superset these exercises due to gym set-up, then perform each separately with 30 seconds of rest between sets.				

Active Recovery Phase #3

DURATION: 1 WEEK

Purpose: Allows for recovery of the body to prime it for the muscle-building phase.

Training Methodology: Fast-paced full body routine consisting largely of dumbbells to allow for maximum involvement of all muscles as well as to correct any strength imbalances in the body.

MONDAY/THURSDAY			FULL BODY ROUTINE	
EXERCISE	PAGE NO.	REPS	SETS	REST
SUPERSET # 1				
Incline Dumbbell Press	74	13-15	2	No Rest
Pulldown to Front (wide grip)	94	13-15	2	1 minute
SUPERSET # 2				
Dumbbell Bench Press	76	13-15	2	No Rest
One Arm Dumbbell Rows	96	13-15	2	1 minute
SUPERSET # 3				
Bent-over Lateral Raises	122	13-15	2	No Rest
Dumbbell Shoulder Press	116	13-15	2	1 minute
SUPERSET # 4				
Incline Dumbbell Curls	140	13-15	2	No Rest
Overhead Dumbbell Triceps Extensions	164	13-15	2	1 minute
SUPERSET # 5				
Squats	177	13-15	2	No Rest
Lying Leg Curls	204	13-15	2	1 minute
SUPERSET # 6				
Leg Extensions	182	13-15	2	No Rest
Standing Calf Raises	218	13-15	2	1 minute
SUPERSET #7				
Lying Leg Raises	240	13-15	2	No Rest
Crunches	238	13-15	2	1 minute

Hybrid Phase: Volume/Strength Training

WEEKS: 16–18

DURATION: 3 WEEKS

Purpose: Allows for a smooth transition from the Volume Phase to the Strength Training Phase. In this phase, muscle growth will occur through an intra-cellular increase of energy substrates and water and also through an increase in the size of the muscle fiber itself.

Training Methodology: You will target and train each body part twice a week. However, the amount of sets per body part will be reduced so that the muscles can recover. The first two days, you will train for hypertrophy while the remaining two days you will train for strength.

MONDAY		CHEST/BACK/BICEPS/TRICEPS/UPPER ABS		
EXERCISE	**PAGE NO.**	**REPS**	**SETS**	**REST**
SUPERSET # 1 Incline Dumbbell Press (adjust bench to an angle of 25 degrees)	74	8–10	3	No Rest
Pull-up to Front (close grip, palms facing forward)	98	8–10	3	1 minute
NOTES: If you cannot perform the pull-up, have your partner assist or use a weight assist machine. Otherwise, substitute pull-downs.				
SUPERSET # 2 Dumbbell Bench Press	76	10–12	3	No Rest
Neutral Grip Pull-Ups	102	10–12	3	1 minute
NOTES: If you cannot perform the pull-up, have your partner assist or use a weight assist machine. Otherwise, substitute pull-downs.				
SUPERSET # 3 Dumbbell Hammer Curls	144	8–10	3	No Rest
Overhead Dumbbell Triceps Extensions	164	8–10	3	1 minute
SUPERSET # 4 Dumbbell Preacher Curls	146	10–12	3	No Rest
Triceps Pushdown	170	10–12	3	1 minute
Crunches	238	15–20	3	1 minute

HARDGAINERS

TUESDAY — THIGHS/HAMSTRINGS/DELTS/CALVES/LOWER ABS

EXERCISE	PAGE NO.	REPS	SETS	REST
SUPERSET # 1				
Squats (wide stance)	177	8–10	3	No Rest
Dumbbell Stiff-Legged Deadlifts	200	8–10	3	1 minute
NOTES: If you suffer from lower back problems, substitute the wide stance squat for a wide stance leg press, and press with toes to target and train your quads.				
SUPERSET # 2				
Leg Extensions	182	10–12	3	No Rest
Lying Leg Curls	204	10–12	3	1 minute
SUPERSET # 3				
Lateral Raises	128	8–10	3	No Rest
Standing Calf Raises	218	8–10	3	1 minute
SUPERSET # 4				
Bent-over Lateral Raises	122	10–12	3	No Rest
Seated Calf Raises	224	10–12	3	1 minute
Hanging Leg Raises	242	10–12	3	1 minute

THURSDAY — CHEST/BACK/BICEPS/TRICEPS

EXERCISE	PAGE NO.	REPS	SETS	REST
MODIFIED COMPOUND SUPERSET # 1				
Incline Barbell Press	78	8, 6, 4	3	90 Seconds
Close-Grip Chins	100	8, 6, 4	3	90 Seconds
NOTES: If you cannot perform the pull-up, have your partner assist or use a weight assist machine. Otherwise, substitute pull-downs.				
MODIFIED COMPOUND SUPERSET # 2				
Chest Dips	80	8, 6, 4	3	90 Seconds
Pull-up to Front (wide grip)	98	8, 6, 4	3	90 Seconds
NOTES: If you cannot perform the pull-up, have your partner assist or use a weight assist machine. Otherwise, substitute pull-downs.				
MODIFIED COMPOUND SUPERSET # 3				
E-Z Curls	148	8, 6, 4	3	60-second rest
Close Grip Bench Press	160	8, 6, 4	3	60-second rest
MODIFIED COMPOUND SUPERSET # 4				
E-Z Preacher Curls	150	8, 6, 4	3	60-second rest
Lying Triceps Extensions	166	8, 6, 4	3	No Rest
Crunches	238	8, 6, 4	3	60-second rest
NOTES: The way this superset is performed is by doing the curls first, resting 60 seconds, moving to the extensions, and then without rest to the crunches. After the crunches, rest 60 seconds and start over.				

FRIDAY — THIGHS/HAMSTRINGS/DELTS/CALVES

EXERCISE	PAGE NO.	REPS	SETS	REST
MODIFIED COMPOUND SUPERSET # 1				
Squats (medium stance)	177	8, 6, 4	3	90 Seconds
Lying Leg Curls	204	8, 6, 4	3	90 Seconds
NOTES: If you suffer from lower back problems you may replace the squat with the leg press. Since you are performing the leg press as your second exercise, use a close stance on this one and a medium stance on the second one.				
MODIFIED COMPOUND SUPERSET # 2				
Quadriceps Leg Press	180	8, 6, 4	3	90 Seconds
Barbell Stiff-Legged Deadlifts	202	8, 6, 4	3	90 Seconds
MODIFIED COMPOUND SUPERSET # 3				
Seated Military Press	118	8, 6, 4	3	60 second rest
Calf Press	220	8, 6, 4	3	60 second rest
MODIFIED COMPOUND SUPERSET # 4				
Upright Rows	120	8, 6, 4	3	60 second rest
Standing Calf Raises	218	10, 8, 6	3	No rest
Lying Leg Raises	240	10, 8, 6	3	60 second rest
NOTES: In order to finish the routine within the allotted time, lying leg raises were included in this last modified compound superset. The way this superset is performed is by doing the upright rows first, resting 60 seconds, moving to the calf raises, and then without rest to the leg raises. After the leg raises, rest 60 seconds and start over.				

HARDGAINERS

Strength Phase (Volume/Strength Training)

DURATION: 3 WEEKS   WEEKS: 19–21

Purpose: To increase muscle size and strength. This is accomplished by loading the muscle with the maximum weight it can handle in order to increase fast-twitch muscle recruitment, and thus increase the protein content of the muscle and the thickness of the muscle fibers.

Training Methodology: You will target and train each body part once a week using modified compound sets. In this phase you will train all your muscles by pairing them with their antagonistic counterparts. Research indicates that pairing opposing muscles together increases the recruitment of the muscle fibers. For example, while during leg training I've found isolating the quads and hamstrings works well during the hypertrophy phases, but during strength phases, pairing the quads and hamstrings provides better results.

We will largely use 5 sets of 5 repetitions, popularized back in the 50s by Mr. Universe Reg Park (Arnold Schwarzenegger's idol). In this method, you choose a weight that allows you to do 5 perfect reps. Your goal is to complete all sets with the same weight at 5 reps. Once you can complete all 5 sets with 5 perfect reps, you increase the weight at the next workout.

MONDAY/THURSDAY				CHEST/BACK
EXERCISE	**PAGE NO.**	**REPS**	**SETS**	**REST**
MODIFIED COMPOUND SUPERSET # 1				
Incline Barbell Press	78	5	5	90 Seconds
Close Grip Chins	100	5	5	90 Seconds
NOTES: If you cannot perform the pull-up, have your partner assist or use a weight assist machine. Otherwise, substitute pull-downs.				
MODIFIED COMPOUND SUPERSET # 2				
Chest Dips	80	5	5	90 Seconds
Pull-up to Front (wide grip)	98	5	5	90 Seconds
NOTES: If you cannot perform the pull-up, have your partner assist or use a weight assist machine. Otherwise, substitute pull-downs.				
Bent Knee Deadlifts (wide stance)	104	5	5	90 Seconds
NOTES: If you have lower back problems, do not include this exercise! If you do, perform with the utmost respect and the most excellent form possible.				

TUESDAY — DELTS/CALVES/UPPER ABS

EXERCISE	PAGE NO.	REPS	SETS	REST
MODIFIED COMPOUND SUPERSET # 1				
Seated Military Press	118	5	5	90 seconds
Upright Rows	120	5	5	90 seconds
MODIFIED COMPOUND SUPERSET # 2				
Calf Press	220	5	5	90 seconds
Tibia Raises	226	25–40	5	90 seconds
Crunches	238	5	5	90 seconds

THURSDAY — BICEPS/TRICEPS/DELTS

EXERCISE	PAGE NO.	REPS	SETS	REST
MODIFIED COMPOUND SUPERSET # 1				
E-Z Reverse Curls	152	5	5	90 seconds
Close Grip Bench Press	160	5	5	90 seconds
MODIFIED COMPOUND SUPERSET # 2				
E-Z Preacher Curls	150	5	5	90 seconds
Triceps Dips	162	5	5	90 seconds

FRIDAY — QUADRICEPS/CALVES/UPPER ABS

EXERCISE	PAGE NO.	REPS	SETS	REST
SUPERSET # 1				
Squats (medium stance)	177	5	5	90 seconds
Lying Leg Curls	204	5	5	90 seconds
NOTES: If you suffer from lower back problems you may substitute the leg press for the squat. Since you are performing the leg press as your second exercise, use a close stance on this one and a medium stance on the second one.				
SUPERSET # 2				
Quadriceps Leg Press	180	5	5	90 seconds
Barbell Stiff-Legged Deadlifts	202	5	5	No rest
Lying Leg Raises	240	5	5	90 seconds

What To Do After Week 21

After week 21 you can loop back to week 1 to go through the entire process again. You may feel free to change exercises or change exercise order; just attempt to stay within the parameters of the program.

What If I Have Limited Equipment

The minimum equipment necessary for this program is a pair of good adjustable dumbbells and an adjustable bench with a leg extension/leg curl attachment. It's extremely important to ensure your equipment is of high quality. Do not run the risk of buying unsafe, cheap equipment and getting injured. While you can buy adjustable dumbbells in any sporting good stores, there are a couple of ingenious dumbbell systems that I would recommend. The first set is the ingenious PowerBlock set, from www.powerblocks.com, which provides the capability to select the weight with only the change of a pin. Depending on the set selected, you can go from 5 lb up to 125! The second set is a more traditional-looking set that is more rugged and secure than the Powerblocks. It is called the IronMaster Quick-Lock Dumbbells, from www.IronMaster.com, and this set can go from 5 lb up to 120 lb. While it takes slightly longer to change the weights, it does provide added security as well as the benefits provided by traditional dumbbells (such as the fact that the wrist is not bound in some motions). I like to use this set for any lifts that go over 50 lb and I reserve my Powerblocks for lifts of 50 lb and below. In that manner I get the best of both worlds.

Another company, Body Solid, manufactures good equipment, like squat racks and heavy-duty Olympic benches, for those of us who prefer working out in a gym at home. You can find their equipment, at a discount, through the Fitness Factory Outlet (www.fitnessfactory.com).

Revisiting the issue of limited equipment, if the only exercise equipment available is a pair of adjustable dumbbells and a good bench, simply replace the exercises discussed with the closest exercise that you can find on the list provided below. In back exercises, unfortunately, only the rows may be substituted for a pull-up. While pull-ups are my personal preference, rows are still an excellent mass building exercise.

Back: One Arm Dumbbell Rows (palms facing your body), Two Arm Dumbbell Rows (palms facing forward as if you were doing regular barbell rows), Two Arm Dumbbell Rows (reverse grip), Bent-Arm Pullovers

Chest: Incline Dumbbell Press (at all angles supported by your bench), Dumbbell Bench Press, Flies (incline and flat)

Thighs: Close, Medium, and Wide Stance Squats (holding each dumbbell by your side), Lunges (all variations such as static, walking, alternating legs, to the side), Sissy Squats, Leg Extensions (all variations—toes in, straight, and out)

Hamstrings: Stiff-Legged Deadlifts, Lying Leg Curls (all variations—toes in, straight, and out)

Shoulders: Shoulder Press, Upright Rows, Lateral Raises, Bent-over Lateral Raises, Bent-over Laterals performed facing down on an incline bench, Bent-over Laterals performed with bent elbows

Traps: Shrugs and Upright Rows

Biceps: Biceps Curls, One Arm Preacher Curls (using the bench in its incline position), Incline Dumbbell Curls, Concentration Curls, Hammer Curls

Triceps: Lying Triceps Extensions, Overhead Triceps Extensions, Close Grip Bench Press, Triceps Kickbacks

Calves: Two-Legged Dumbbell Calf Raises & One-Legged Dumbbell Calf Raises

Abdominals: Crunches, Bicycle Crunches, Lying Leg Raises, Knee-Ins, V-Ups

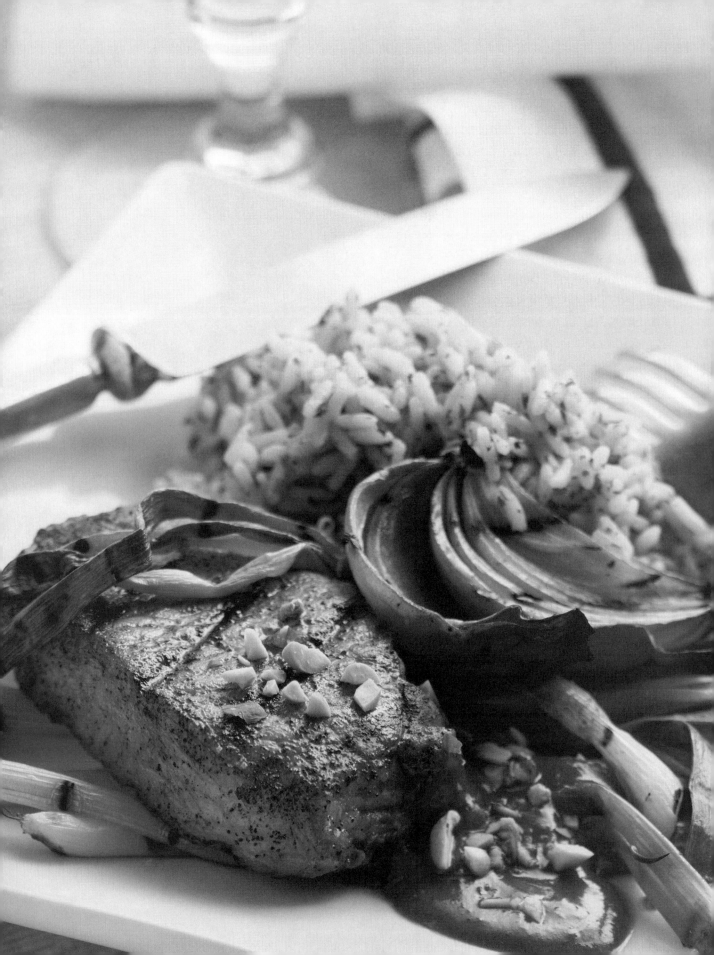

CHAPTER 4
Mass Building Nutrition

The wheel is in motion to get you the body of your dreams. You have set your goal for the future, examined the formula for muscle growth success, and reviewed the exercise plan you will follow. Now, it's time to discuss the component of the muscle growth formula that the hardgainer needs to understand the most: nutrition. As I have previously mentioned, hardgainers have a very fast metabolism, and if not fed properly, the hardgainer can never expect to gain any appreciable muscle.

In order for hardgainers to gain muscle mass, they need to take in more calories than their bodies burn on any given day. When your caloric intake exceeds your body's metabolic requirements, you enter a state of anabolism: a state where food particles are synthesized into complex living tissue such as muscle and fat.

Having said that, is it possible to gain muscle without gaining any body fat? Is it possible to enter a state of anabolism where only muscle, and not fat, is gained? Unlikely, unless you fall under one of the following conditions:

- You are a beginner in which case you gain muscle and can even lose body fat at the same time as the stimulus provided by weight training is a completely new thing for your body.
- You are regaining muscle that you have lost due to sickness or inactivity.
- You are taking enormous amounts of steroids and thyroid hormone.

If you do not fall under one of these three categories, then your goal is not to eliminate body fat, but to gain muscle while maintaining the same level of body fat or minimize its increase. You accomplish this by ensuring that the calories taken in are high quality calories your body will likely use for recovery and muscle repair as opposed to fat storage. This brings us to the next section that will teach you what macronutrients you should be eating on a daily basis. You will also learn what amounts are required in order to maximize muscle growth and minimize fat loss.

Nutrition Basics

There are 3 macronutrients that the human body needs in order to function properly: carbohydrates, protein, and fat. In addition, a healthy quantity of water is required.

Carbohydrates

Carbohydrates are your body's main source of energy. When you ingest carbohydrates, your pancreas releases a hormone called insulin, which:

- Chemically bonds to carbohydrates and stores them in the muscle or as fat.
- Chemically bonds to amino acids (protein) and shelters them inside the muscle cell for recovery and repair.

In short, insulin holds the key to carbohydrate metabolism (energy production), protein synthesis (muscle production), and fat synthesis (storage of carbs, protein, and fats as fat tissue).

Because of their fast metabolisms, hardgainers require an abundance of carbs (around 50% of their total caloric intake). Such a large carbohydrate requirement ensures their bodies' amino acid supply is not used as a source of energy. If your body burns all the carbs available in the muscles and liver (glycogen) as well as the ones ingested, then the next step is to burn amino acids (muscle) as well as fat. Since most hardgainers do not have a large carbohydrate base, nor big amounts of body fat, they burn muscle for energy and as a result do not grow muscle.

Carbohydrates are divided into two categories: complex and simple. Complex carbs give you sustained energy ("timed release"), while simple carbs give you immediate energy. For hardgainers, I recommend that an equal amount of complex and simple carbohydrates be consumed throughout the day. The hardgainer has such a fast metabolism that he requires more simple carbs than ordinarily consumed to keep fueling his metabolism. While this strategy would cause a typical endomorph with a slow metabolism to get fat, this helps keep the hardgainer from losing hard-earned muscle.

Simple carbs are great to ingest during the first 20 to 30 minutes following a workout, when they will be immediately needed to replenish glycogen levels in your body. After a workout, it is in your best interest to raise insulin levels sharply to take full advantage of the post-workout window of opportunity. During this 20- to 30-minute window, the body is more interested in using nutrients for muscle repair and production than for fat storage. At this time, eating simple carbohydrates that are released quickly into the blood stream helps to speed up recuperation and aid in the production of lean muscle tissue.

Below is a list of good carbohydrate sources.

COMPLEX CARBOHYDRATES:

There are two types of complex carbohydrates. You should be eating these complex carbs in your breakfast, lunch, and dinner.

- **Starchy:** oatmeal, potatoes, grits, brown rice, lentils, sweet potatoes, whole wheat bread, cream of rice, chickpeas, and pitas
- **Fibrous:** asparagus, squash, broccoli, green beans, cabbage, cauliflower, celery, cucumber, mushrooms, lettuce, red or green peppers, tomato, spinach, and zucchini

SIMPLE CARBOHYDRATES:

Good sources of simple carbs are:

- bananas, grapes, skim milk (also contains protein), strawberries, apples, pears, cantaloupes, cherries, grapefruit, lemon, nectarine, peaches

Protein

Every tissue in your body is made up of protein (muscles, hair, skin, nails, etc.). Protein is the building block of lean muscle tissue. Without it, building muscle and burning fat would be impossible. Protein helps increase your metabolism every time you digest it by up to 20 percent, and it releases carbohydrates (glucose) slowly throughout the day, resulting in higher energy levels.

For the purposes of this program, you will begin to consume 1.5 grams of protein per pound of bodyweight (this is around 25% of your total caloric intake). This amount of protein will ensure that you have more than enough amino acids in your system for repair and rebuilding of muscle tissue.

Good examples of protein include: salmon, halibut, cod, round steak, chicken breast, tuna fish (springwater), sardines, turkey breast, whey protein, egg substitutes, and skim milk (which also contains simple carbs and ideally should be limited to post workout or in between meals).

Fats

All the cells in the body have some fat. Fats are responsible for the lubrication of your joints. In addition, many hormones are manufactured from fats. If you eliminate all fat from your diet, your hormonal production will drop and many chemical reactions necessary to keep your body functioning will be interrupted. Your body will begin to accumulate more body fat to keep functioning. Because your testosterone production is halted, the production of lean muscle mass will be halted as well. Looking back at this chain reaction, it's easy to come to the conclusion that to have an efficient metabolism, we need to consume certain fats.

There are three types of fats: saturated, polyunsaturated, and monounsaturated.

- **Saturated Fats:** Saturated fats are associated with heart disease and high cholesterol levels. To a large extent, they are found in products of animal origin. However, some vegetable fats are altered by hydrogenation and thus also have a high level of saturated fat. Generally found in packaged foods, these hydrogenated vegetable oils include coconut oil, palm oil, and palm kernel oil. Non-dairy creamers are also a culprit.

• **Polyunsaturated Fats:** These fats do not have an effect on cholesterol levels. The majority of the fats in vegetable oils, such as corn, cottonseed, safflower, soybean, and sunflower oil, are polyunsaturated. In addition, flaxseed oil and fish oils are polyunsaturated and are unusually high in omega-3 essential fatty acids (EFAs), one of the two essential fats that the body needs. The body is unable to produce them on its own and omega-3 EFAs must be obtained from the diet. The second EFA the body requires is omega-6. While flax and fish oils also contain to a lesser extent the omega-6, these fats are found abundantly in egg and poultry. Both essential fats improve the immune system, energy production, insulin sensitivity, and hormonal production. Omega-3 in particular, have been also shown to have anti-lipogenic properties and help prevent fat storage, as well as assisting to burn body fat, and improving recovery. The omega-6, on the other hand, have been shown to have anti-inflammatory properties which protect muscle from being broken down, and are also beneficial to the body by also reducing post training inflammation. These oils, however, are easily found in most vegetable oils, margarine, poultry, and eggs, so omega-6 supplements are unnecessary.

• **Monounsaturated Fats:** These fats have a positive effect on good cholesterol levels. Sources of these fats are virgin olive oil, canola oil, and peanut oil.

While I typically do not recommend more than 20% fats for most people, hardgainers tend to benefit with a fat intake as high as 25%. For the purposes of this book, 25% of your calories should come from good fats, preferably an even split between flaxseed (preferably organic whole ground flaxseed) or fish oils, plus extra virgin olive oil and natural peanut butter. Add to this naturally occurring animal fats from lean meats and whole eggs, and this should provide you with saturated fat from good sources. Some saturated fat is needed for hormonal production, so it is not wise to entirely cut saturated fat from your diet.

Water

Water is by far the most abundant substance in our body. Without water, no one could survive for very long. Most people that are looking for advice on how to get in shape underestimate the value of water.

• Over 65% of your body is composed of water.

• Water cleanses your body of toxins and pollutants that can make you sick.

• A lack of water would interrupt processes such as energy production, muscle building, and fat burning.

• Water lubricates the joints, resulting in increased mobility and decreased joint pain.

• When the outside temperature increases, water cools the body, bringing its temperature down to where it is supposed to be.

• Water helps control your appetite. Have

you ever felt like you were still hungry after eating a huge meal? This might very well be an indication that your body is beginning to dehydrate. You will notice that by drinking water at that time, your cravings will stop.

• Cold water increases your metabolism and aids in the breakdown of brown body fat.

In order to determine how much water your body needs each day, multiply your lean body weight by .66. This indicates how many ounces of water your body requires in a day for optimal function.

The Importance of Multiple Meals

Multiple meals throughout the day are extremely important. If you neglect to feed your body, waiting over three or four hours until your next meal, your body switches to a catabolic state in which your body uses fat and muscle tissue for energy. The body believes that it is starving, and in an attempt to protect itself, begins to feed by cannibalizing both your muscle and fat tissue.

Another reason to eat frequent meals is to keep your blood sugar, insulin management, and energy levels steady. Larger infrequent feedings result in larger releases of insulin with blood sugar crashes, resulting in low energy levels 30 minutes to an hour after the meal was eaten. In addition, extra calories the body cannot use at that time are stored for future use as body fat. A low blood sugar level will make you lethargic and

you may have cravings for sweets. Smaller, more frequent feedings spike the metabolism and maintain a more stable blood sugar pattern that results in better use of nutrients, more stable energy, and reduced cravings throughout the day.

The Rules of Anabolic Nutrition

In order for you to begin on the path to muscle growth, you will have to set up an individualized plan to create your anabolic environment. Anabolic refers to a metabolic condition in which new molecules are synthesized (created) from simple ones; such as when the body uses food (simple molecules) to create new muscle (new molecules). To create an anabolic environment, we provide a stimulus to the body that gives it a need to create new muscle. We do this through weight training. Then, through an increased intake of food, we provide the raw materials needed to build the new muscle tissue.

So having said that, in order to create an anabolic environment that is conductive to growth we need to:

Calculate a caloric intake that covers your basal metabolic rate and activity level. I want you to take your body weight and multiply it by 24. For example, if you weigh 150 lb, then 150 x 24 = 3600. This will be your starting caloric intake. If you gain 1 lb your first week of eating this many calories, then maintain this level. A weight gain of less than a pound will require a further increase of 240 calories.

Calculate the grams of protein that you will require on your diet. To calculate this, you will need to multiply your body weight times 1.5. So, continuing with the example of the 150-lb bodybuilder, 150 x 1.5 = 225 grams of protein; which comes out to 900 calories (225 grams of protein x 4 calories per gram = 900 calories). This much protein will not affect kidney function; as a matter of fact, there is no research that indicates that a high protein diet affects healthy kidney function. I have been following high protein diets for over fifteen years now and when I last checked my blood work, there was no indication that my kidneys have been stressed (and I have increased my protein intake at some points to 3 grams of protein per pound of body weight). Having said this, it is important to note that if you suffer from kidney problems, a high protein diet may not be suitable for you as in this case the extra protein may place further stress on the organ. Also, let's remember the importance of drinking plenty of water (at least your body weight times .66 in ounces of water per day), as a lack of water combined with a high protein diet does place stress on the kidneys.

Calculate the amounts of good fats that you will need. As mentioned above, hardgainers should get 25% of their calories from good fats. So for the 150-lb bodybuilder, a fat intake of body weight x 0.666 will yield around 100 grams of fat, which accounts for 900 calories (100 grams of fat x 9 calories per gram = 900 calories). From these 100 grams, we'll separate 30 grams for saturated, 35 for monounsaturated (olive oil and peanut butter) and 35 for polyunsaturated (fish oils and flax seed source).

Calculate the amounts of carbohydrates that you will need. The carbohydrate calculation is simple. Bodyweight x 3 equals the grams of carbohydrates you need. Therefore, the 150-lb bodybuilder needs 150 x 3 = 450 grams of carbohydrates which accounts for 1800 calories (450 grams of carbohydrates x 4). Since we have six meals in one day, I would like you to split your carbohydrates equally into simple carbs and complex carbs, so 225 grams will come from simple sources and the other 225 grams will be complex. Simple sources should be used for the post workout meal and for in between breakfast, lunch, and dinner, while complex carbs will be used during the three main meals. It is also a good idea to add fibrous sources in the middle of the day and at night as they help in protein digestion and processing. Anywhere between 10 and 15 grams is acceptable.

Space out all nutrients in 6 meals per day. We know that our 150-lb bodybuilder needs around 225 grams of protein per day. This works out to be about 37.5 grams of protein per meal. If you want to, you can round that off to 40 grams. So each of your six meals needs at least 37.5 grams of protein. Dividing 450 by 6 yields for 75 grams of carbohydrates. Finally, fat requirements of 100 grams divided by six yields around 17 grams. However, for the after workout meal, it's suggested to have no fats, as that nutrient will slow down the release of carbohydrates into the muscle, which the muscle will need badly at that time. Instead of dividing by six, I would like you to divide fats by five, so that you can modify your diet for the workout days. This would yield 20 grams of fat in each of five meals.

The Rules in Choosing Foods:

• Always try to use natural foods. Avoid using canned or prepared foods as they usually contain excessive amounts of fat, sodium and sugar.

• Stay within plus or minus 10 grams of the recommended amount of carbs and proteins. Remember to keep fats to a minimum.

• Always choose low-fat protein sources. If you eat extremely low-fat meals, don't worry about incurring a fat deficiency because the supplements program will take care of essential fatty acids. There are also trace amounts of fat even in the low-fat protein sources that you may choose.

• If you choose to include skim milk in your diet, remember that it not only has protein (8 to 9 grams for every 8 ounces of milk) but also simple carbs (12 to 13 grams for every 8 ounces of milk). Therefore, count milk as both.

• Try to include fibrous carbs in at least two meals.

What To Eat And When

Now that you know how to figure out your individual nutrient needs, let's look at how to set up your meal plan, and also what sorts of foods to choose from.

In the tables below, there are lists of foods that you can choose from in order to create your meals. Each item listed contains the gram amounts they provide of each nutrient we have discussed.

Meal Plan Schedule

Using the calculations from the previous section create a diet using the foods from the table above. Your meal plan will consist of breakfast, lunch, and dinner with three snacks in between. The snacks can be in the form of real food or protein shakes (your choice). In order to develop your meal plan you will need to first calculate all of your daily requirements of protein, carbohydrates and fat. Then divide your requirements into 6 and fill in the gram requirements in the menu list below.

Notes: I based the schedule on an 8 a.m.–5 p.m. job but you can modify it to suit your individual situation. If you workout at any other time than the evening then just move the post workout meal to the time at which you are done working out and continue with the next meal following. For instance, if you work out at 10 a.m. then your post workout meal will be at 11 or 11: 30 a.m. (the latest) and then the following meal will be your lunch 2 to 3 hours later. The mid-morning snack then will become your late evening snack to be consumed around 9 p.m.

FOOD GROUP TABLES

MEAL 1 *(7:00 a.m.)*   **BREAKFAST**

Choose _____ grams from Group A
Choose _____ grams from Group B
Choose _____ grams from Group E

MEAL 2 *(10:00 a.m.)*   **MID-MORNING**

Choose _____ grams from Group A
Choose _____ grams from Group C
Choose _____ grams from Group E

MEAL 3 *(12:30 p.m.)*   **LUNCH**

Choose _____ grams from Group A
Choose _____ grams from Group B
Choose _____ grams from Group D
Choose _____ grams from Group E

MEAL 4 *(3:00 p.m.)*   **MID-AFTERNOON**

Choose _____ grams from Group A
Choose _____ grams from Group C
Choose _____ grams from Group E

MEAL 5 *(5:30 p.m.)*   **EARLY DINNER**

Choose _____ grams from Group A
Choose _____ grams from Group B
Choose _____ grams from Group D
Choose _____ grams from Group E

WORKOUT:7:30PM—8:30PM

MEAL 5 *(9:00 p.m.)*   **POST WORKOUT MEAL**

Choose _____ grams from Group A
Choose _____ grams from Group C

GROUP A - PROTEIN

FOOD	GRAMS	FOOD	GRAMS
Chicken breast (3.5 oz broiled)	33	White fish (3.5 oz broiled)	31
Tuna (packed in water, 3.5 oz)	35	Halibut (3.5 oz broiled)	31
Turkey breast (3.5 oz broiled)	28	Cod (3.5 oz broiled)	31
Whey protein powder (2 scoops)	22	Round steak (3.5 oz broiled)	33
10 egg whites	35	Top sirloin (4 oz)	35

Note: These weights are for uncooked portions

GROUP B - CARBOHYDRATE (COMPLEX, STARCHY)

FOOD	GRAMS	FOOD	GRAMS
Baked potato (3.5 oz broiled)	21	Lentils (1 cup dry, cooked)	38
Plain oatmeal (1/2 cup dry)	27	Grits (1/4 cup dry)	31
Whole wheat bread	13	Chickpeas (1 cup cooked)	45
(limit if trying to go below 10% body fat		Brown rice (2/3 cup cooked)	30
as wheat contains pythoestrogens)		Cream of Rice (1/4 cup dry, post workout only)	38
Pita bread (1 piece)	33	Sweet potato (4 oz)	28

GROUP C - CARBOHYDRATE (SIMPLE)

FOOD	GRAMS	FOOD	GRAMS
Apple (1)	15	Banana (6 oz, post workout only)	27
Cantaloupe (1/2)	25	Grapes (1 cup, post workout only)	14
Strawberries (1 cup)	9	Grapefruit (1/2)	12
Orange (1)	15	Tangerine (1)	9
Pear (1)	27	Cherries (1 cup)	22
Lemon (1)	5	Nectarine (1)	16
Peach (1)	10	Skim milk (1 cup, preferably post workout only)	13

GROUP D - CARBOHYDRATE (COMPLEX, FIBROUS)

FOOD (10 oz serving)	GRAMS	FOOD (10 oz serving)	GRAMS
Asparagus	5	Yellow squash	12
Broccoli	17	Green beans	23
Cabbage	6	Cauliflower	12
Celery	6	Cucumber	7
Mushrooms	6	Lettuce	7
Red or green peppers	15	Tomato	5
Spinach	3	Zucchini	13

GROUP E - GOOD FATS

MONOUNSATURATED (1 TABLESPOON)	GRAMS	POLYUNSATURATED (1 TABLESPOON)	GRAMS
Extra virgin olive oil	14	Flaxseed oil	14
Natural peanut butter	8	Fish oils	14

Anabolic Nutrition Summary

I know that at first it can be overwhelming to create your muscle gain nutrition plan. In this section I will go over it again, so that in a few easy steps you are on your way to a bigger, more muscular physique:

STEP 1: CALCULATE YOUR CALORIC INTAKE.

Body weight x 24 = Total number of calories required per day

STEP 2: CALCULATE YOUR DAILY NUTRIENT REQUIREMENTS.

Since we follow a ratio of:

50 % Carbohydrates

25 % Proteins

25 % Good fats

We acquire the daily grams by using the formulas below:

Total grams of carbs for the day =
(Total number of calories x 0.50)/4

Total grams of protein for the day =
(Total number of calories x 0.25)/4

Total grams of fat for the day =
(Total number of calories x 0.25)/9

-or-

You can use the simpler formulas below:

Total grams of carbs for the day =
Body weight in pounds x 3

Total grams of protein for the day =
Body weight in pounds x 1.5

Total grams of fat for the day =
Body weight in pounds x 0.666

If this is too cumbersome, do not worry. In Appendix A, I already have all of these calculations for you on a matrix, so just find out your weight and the matrix will tell you the amount of calories and nutrients you need per day.

STEP 3: CALCULATE YOUR NUTRIENT REQUIREMENTS PER MEAL.

Divide each macronutrient requirement in grams by six in order to determine the amount needed per meal. For fats on training days, remember to just divide by five as we do not want to take in fats in the post workout meal.

STEP 4: PLUG IN THE VALUES IN THE MEAL PLAN SCHEDULE FROM APPENDIX B.

STEP 5: CHOOSE THE DESIRED FOODS BY USING THE FOOD GROUP TABLES FROM APPENDIX C.

Use Appendix D to write down your food items and the quantity of each.

Troubleshooting Your Caloric Intake

A good rate of bulking up is 1 to 2 lb per week. Any more than 2 lb and you can risk putting on too much body fat. If you do not gain at least 1 lb after your first week of training and dieting, then increase your calories by 240. To make things easier on you, the best way to recalculate the nutrients is to go back to Appendix A. For instance, if you were using the values for the 150 lb person (assuming that you are a 150-lb bodybuilder) then use the values for the 160 lb bodybuilder on the following week. If you gain at least 1 lb then stay at that level until you cease to make gains. If you still miss the 1-lb mark, then increase again to the values of the 170-lb bodybuilder.

If on the other hand, at the current level you gain 4 lb and you notice that your physique is looking softer due to the fact that you are gaining too much fat, then back off by reducing 240 calories in the form of carbohydrates. So if you were on the 150-lb plan, and take in 450 grams of carbohydrates throughout the day, then you need to eliminate 60 grams of carbohydrates per day (240 divided by 4 equals 60) in order to harden up. So all you have to do then is reduce each meal carbohydrate intake by 10 grams and you will be on your way to a harder looking you. This is, by the way, the manner in which competitive bodybuilders achieve very low levels of bodyfat. If you want to harden up even more, then every couple of weeks reduce calories in this manner. However, do not go below the point in which protein grams and carbohydrate grams are equal.

There is no need to decrease calories if you are gaining muscle and definition is hardly affected (this is even if you gain 5 lb). However, if you are getting softer looking then it is better to drop slightly to assure that most gains come in the form of muscle and not fat.

Cooking Tips

If you want to achieve your goals, proper food preparation is essential! Follow the guidelines below to ensure proper food preparation:

- Eat vegetables raw or slightly steamed. If boiling, be careful not to overcook or you will lose the nutritional value of the vegetables.
- Do not fry. Always broil, grill, steam or bake (broiling, grilling and steaming are better as they allow fat to drain while cooking).
- Trim all fat from meat and remove skin from poultry prior to cooking.
- Do not use salts, butter, oils, or sugar while cooking. Experiment with herbs, non-salt seasonings, lemon juice, vinegar, garlic and pepper, even a touch (1 tbsp.; not a bottle) of some white or red wine. Occasional use of salsa, low-sodium soy sauce, catsup, and mustard to enhance meats and vegetables is OK if used sparingly (1 tbsp.). Minced white or green onions are also excellent for seasoning.

The Hardgainer's Best Ally: Food Preparation and the Cooler

The best thing you can do for yourself is to go out and buy a cooler and a whole bunch of containers to carry your food with you. As you can see, your results will be tied to your capacity to get frequent meals throughout the day. For this reason, preparation is crucial to the success of your dietary program. If you are not prepared, you will fail!

Beverage Tips

Beware!!! You can eat the most nutritious food in the world and still blow your diet without realizing your doing it! The culprit? Drinking the wrong types of beverages.

- Drink plenty of water daily. Your recommended fluid intake should be 0.66 x body weight in ounces per day.
- Absolutely no regular sodas. For example, the average soda contains 40 grams of sugar!
- Crystal Lite beverages, and decaffeinated tea/coffee are OK as long as they are used in moderation; your main beverage should be water.
- Avoid all alcohol as it lowers testosterone levels and it is great for accumulating fat!

What I suggest is that you prepare the next day's meals either the night before or early the next morning. Store them in the individual food containers and pack them all in the cooler. When the time comes to eat, all I have to do is open up my cooler and choose my corresponding meal, which is ready for me in one of the containers. Also, always take your 50-ounce water bottle everywhere you go. No need to dehydrate and die at work or anywhere else. When you get home, take out the container for dinner, re-heat it, eat it and prepare the food for the following day (after washing the containers, of course).

If you think you will be able to stick to the plan without being prepared, believe me, you are in for a surprise. You will either end up eating the wrong kinds of food, or missing meals. You will definitely end up spending more money because eating out is not cheap.

Therefore, remember to be prepared!

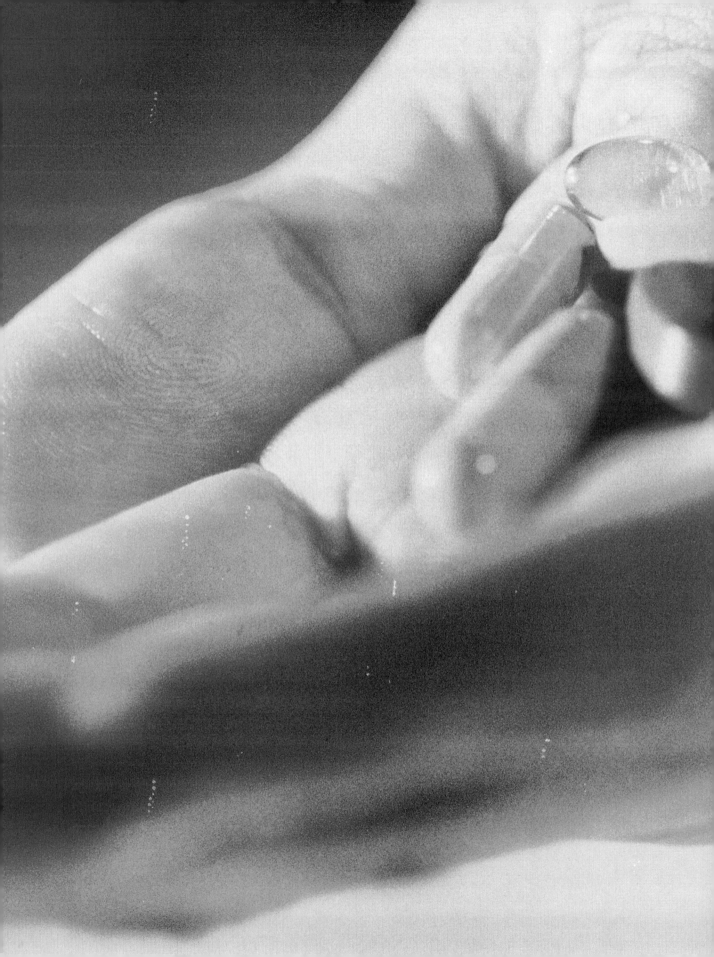

CHAPTER 5
Supplementation For Maximum Growth

Many people incorrectly believe supplements are the most important part of gaining muscle. However, supplements are simply additions to a good nutrition and training program. Supplements do not make up for improper training, or lack thereof, and a crappy diet. Supplements only work when your diet and your training program are optimized.

Nutritional supplements protect us from nutritional deficiencies. Your new exercise programs' increased activity levels make your body require greater amounts of vitamins and minerals, and increase the chances of suffering a nutritional deficiency without supplementation. Remember, even a slight nutrient deficiency can sabotage your muscle growth.

Unfortunately, we cannot rely solely on food to provide us with all the vitamins and minerals that our bodies require. This is largely because of the processing food goes through even before they arrive at the supermarket: cooking, air, and light have already robbed your foods of the vitamins that they normally offer. If you are deficient in one or more essential nutrients, your body may not be able to build muscle and burn fat properly.

However, not all supplements are equal. The use of supplements depends on both your goals and your budget. In the following chapter, I have described the different categories of supplements and have discussed which ones you will need to use at all times.

BASIC SUPPLEMENTS
These basic supplements you will need year round to hit your muscle building goals. If your budget is on the low end, these should be the only supplements you should concern yourself with.

MULTIPLE VITAMIN AND MINERAL FORMULA

This type of supplement is essential to insure that our bodies operate at maximum efficiency. On a very simplistic level, without these vitamins and minerals, it is impossible to covert the food we eat into hormones, tissues, and energy.

Vitamins are organic compounds (produced by both animals and vegetables), that enhance the actions of proteins, causing reactions such as muscle building, fat burning, and energy production. There are two types of vitamins:

- **Fat-soluble vitamins** (such as A, D, E, and K) **are stored in fat and if taken in excessive amounts will become toxic.**
- **Water soluble vitamins are not stored in the body** (such as B-complex and Vitamin C).

Minerals are inorganic compounds not produced by animals or vegetables. Minerals assure that your brain receives the correct signals from the body. Minerals are also involved in regulating the balance of fluids in the body as well as the creation of muscular contractions and energy production. For instance, a calcium, magnesium, and potassium deficiency would cause you to not only have muscle cramps but also have difficulties in contracting your muscles as the ability of the nervous system to transmit signals from the brain will be compromised. Minerals are also necessary for the building of muscle and bones. There are two types of minerals:

- **Bulk minerals, which are called such because the body requires them in great quantities—often in the measure of grams** (such as calcium, magnesium, potassium, sodium and phosphorus).
- **Trace minerals are required by the body in tiny amounts, usually in the order of micrograms** (such as chromium, copper, cobalt, silicon, selenium, iron, and zinc).

WHERE CAN YOU GET THESE VITAMINS AND MINERALS?

I tend to get most of my vitamins and minerals from multiple vitamin/mineral packs. The ones I personally use are the Prolab's Training Paks, which are loaded with potent levels of essential nutrients and bioactive compounds, and Beverly International's Super Pak. I alternate using one for a month and another the following month.

You must be very careful with the vitamin and mineral formula you choose. Some don't always contain what the labels claim, and some come from poor sources and are not absorbed very well by the body. Keeping that in mind, try to stick to this tried-and- true recommended formula list below. Other reputable companies include Twinlabs, EAS, Weider, Labrada, Shiff, Optimum Nutrition, Advanced Nutrition, and Champion Nutrition.

- the Super Spectrum Vitamin/Mineral formula (available at Dave Draper's site: www.davedraper.com)
- Vitamin Shoppes' Health & Fitness Nutrients For Active People (Vitamin Paks)
- GNC's Ultra Mega
- Country Life's Multi-100
- Ultra Two by Nature's Plus

Protein Supplements

It is nearly impossible in today's world to eat six perfectly balanced meals required to get in shape daily. Thus, these supplements can be used as "fast food." They are easy to prepare and the formulas that are available on the market today are as good as a milkshake from any fast food chain. There are many categories of protein supplements, but first let's talk about the different sources of protein found in these supplements.

PROTEIN SOURCES AND *BV* VALUES

Each source of protein is measured by its quality. The measure of the quality of a protein is called Biological Value (BV). BV measures how well the body absorbs and uses the protein, and the higher the BV, the more nitrogen your body can absorb, use, and retain. As a result, proteins with the highest BV promote the most lean muscle gains. Whey protein ranks with the highest BV value, a 104. Egg protein is second with 100, and milk proteins come in third at 91. Beef protein rates an 80 and soy proteins 74. Because bean proteins are plant-based protein, they rank at 49.

Whey Proteins (Whey concentrate/whey isolate). Whey proteins are a great protein source for the following reasons proven by a growing number of studies:

- Improving sports performance by reducing stress and lowering cortisol levels (a hormone that destroys muscle).
- Improving immunity by increasing glutathione (GSH), a water-soluble antioxidant found in the body.
- Improving liver function in some forms of hepatitis
- Reducing blood pressure
- Possibly helping fight HIV
- Helping reduce overtraining (which is linked also to low levels of GSH)

Whey proteins are also highly digestible and have a better amino acid profile than even egg whites. However, whey is not the steroid-like substance magazines are hyping, but based on the research and on my own use of the product, it is a valuable addition to your diet.

Not all whey is created equal. The whey that gives you the benefits described above has to be micro-filtered at very low temperatures to allow production of high protein contents with no undenatured protein, minimum fat, minimum cholesterol, and minimum lactose.

There are also whey isolates and whey concentrates. Whey isolates are sub-fractions of whey absorbed rapidly into the system. While excellent for post workout nutrition, whey isolate is a poor choice for supplementation during the day because if the body does not need all the amino acids released into the bloodstream, it will use them for energy production, not muscle building. Whey isolate also does not have many of the health enhancing properties, as the process required to produce whey isolate destroys many of the health/immune system enhancing sub-fractions. In conclusion, for during the day use, a product consisting mainly of whey concentrate is your best bet, while for after the workout, a whey isolate product will be a better choice.

Egg Protein is a super bio-available protein second only to whey. It is a slower released protein than whey, which makes it perfect for during the day use. I often mix egg and whey protein for one of the most bio-available protein shakes available.

Milk Proteins (calcium caseinate/micellar casein). Similar to egg proteins, these are a highly bio-available protein source, with slightly less BV than the egg equivalent, designed to slowly release into the blood stream. The natural, undenatured protein in milk is micellar casein. Using ultrafiltration and no chemicals, it is isolated in order to increase the bioactive milk peptides that support your immune functions and enhance muscle growth. Micellar casein also may provide a steady release of amino acids, making it an excellent choice for a long-lasting muscle protecting protein.

Beef Proteins are slow released proteins that rate an 80 on the BV scale. While I am unaware of any protein supplement in powder form on the market that is derived from beef proteins, there are beef liver tablets. Beef proteins are rich in blood-building iron and also B-vitamins, both factors that contribute to better nutrient use and energy production.

Soy Proteins have positive health benefits for both men and women. Studies show they may reduce the risk of hormone-dependent cancers (breast, prostate, etc), and possibly protect from other cancers as well. Soy has been well known to reduce high cholesterol and ease the symptoms of menopause. Soy also helps prevent osteoporosis by building up bone mass. Because of this, I recommend one serving of soy protein per day for women, but only for its health benefits. In the muscle building department, soy is not very useful; its BV value is a distant 49, and because it has estrogen-like substances, it might reduce testosterone use, and for men, could be anti-constructive.

PROTEIN SUPPLEMENTS ON MARKET

Now that you have an understanding of the various proteins available in protein supplements, let's discuss the different types of protein supplements on the market.

Weight Gainers are protein shakes consisting mainly of whey proteins. Some also include milk or egg proteins. Characterized by their extremely high carbohydrate content, weight gainers were very popular back in the 90s but their popularity has died mainly because many people do not have the metabolism of a hardgainer, and a high carbohydrate diet leads quickly to fat gains rather than muscle mass gains. For the hardgainer metabolism, these products are very useful for getting the quality calories needed to gain muscle.

The carbohydrate content is designed for a fast release, and is best in the mid-morning, mid-afternoon, and post workout meals. Weight gainers can be mixed with fruit juice or skim milk, and if you are trying to increase the calorie content, adding flaxseed oil and fruits is useful. In Appendix E, we include some sample shakes that show how you can take a product and increase its caloric value to suit your purposes. Some suggested weight gainers on the market are:

- Prolab's N-Large II
- Beverly International's Mass Maker
- Twinlab's Gainers Fuel 2500
- Champion Nutrition's Heavyweight Gainer 900
- Weider's Mega Mass 4000
- Clark Bartram's X-Treme Size
- EAS Mass Factor

This is not a comprehensive list by any means, but rather a list of the products that I know personally. If a product is not on this list, it does not mean that it is not a good one.

Meal Replacement Powders (MRPs) These powders, created after manufacturers realized most of the population did not have a weight gain problem, are lower in calories and have far fewer carbohydrates than weight gainers.

Most powders are composed of whey proteins, but there are many new formulas now on the market that consist of a protein blend of whey and milk proteins. The carbohydrate component used to be maltodextrin, with 25 to 27 grams of carbohydrate per serving, but the new generation of formulas uses slow-release carbohydrates like brown rice and oats to make the product lower in glycemic value. Essential fatty acids and a vitamin and mineral profile have also been added.

While these products have generally too low a calorie count for most hardgainers, this shakes can be used as long as other ingredients such as fruit, skim milk, and essential fats are added. My preferred MRP on the market is Prolab's Lean Mass Matrix; it is instant (all it requires is liquid and a spoon) and has a unique cinnamon oatmeal flavor. My other favorite MRP is Beverly International's Ultra Size as it allows me to manipulate the serving size as it comes with a scoop. It also has a different matrix of proteins than the Lean Mass Matrix so for variety reasons I alternate back and forth between the two. Other recommended products are:

- Champion Nutrition's Ultramet
- EAS's Myoplex
- Labrada's Lean Body

For hardgainers my recommendation is to use weight gainers instead of MRP. If you choose to use these, use them in the same manner as the weight gainers, and make sure you increase the caloric base with the addition of skim milk, essential fats, and fruits.

Protein Powders are powders that consist mainly of protein (typically whey protein, but you can also find blends). They typically contain no more than 5 grams of carbohydrates and 20 to 25 grams of protein per scoop. Calorie-wise, they could be anywhere from 100 to 125 calories. Good sources of these powders are:

- Prolab's Pure Whey
- EAS's MyoPro
- Next Nutrition Designer Protein
- IronTek's Essential Protein

These powders are mainly whey protein concentrate. If you're looking for an isolate, the best on the market are Natures Best Zero Carb Isopure and Prolab's Isolate. The best blends in the market (whey proteins mixed with slower released proteins) are Beverly International's Muscle Provider (whey and egg blend), Dave Draper's Bomber Blend (found through www.davedraper .com), and Prolab's Protein Component (also available in Cinnamon Oatmeal).

The hardgainer can use this powder either to increase the protein content of a weight gainer, or to add protein to a homemade weight gain shake. For bodybuilders on a budget the best way to go sometimes is to buy a 5-lb tub of protein powder and create a home made weight gain formula (see Appendix E).

Protein Bars. These are bars made out of any of the protein sources mentioned above. The carbohydrate mix usually is a combination of glycerin (sugar alcohol, and not really a carbohydrate) and sugars. Bars are low in calories compared to the normal weight gain shake and generally contain fats, which are less than desirable. Use these bars only in cases of extreme emergency when there is nothing better available to eat. The better choices in the market today are:

- Premiere 1 Odyssey Bars
- Chef Jay's Tri-O-Plex Bars
- Labrada's Lean Body Bars
- Met Rx Protein Plus Food Bars
- Labrada's Lean Body Bars
- EAS's Myoplex Deluxe Bars

Beef Liver Tablets are a great source of beef liver, and bodybuilders have been using them for decades. For liver tablets to be useful they have to be manufactured with the highest grade of beef

liver available, and purified of the fat, cholesterol and other impurities in the liver. In my opinion, the best liver tablets on the market are Beverly International's Ultra 40. They contain the highest grade of beef liver and have been purified and processed to contain forty-five times the nutritional amount of whole beef liver. To use these, simply add 3 or 4 tablets per meal. For nutritional purposes, treat each tablet as adding an additional 2 grams of protein from beef liver.

Good Oils

In the nutrition chapter we have already discussed the importance of good fats in your diet. There are four oils that we need to be concerned with: fish oils and flaxseed oil (polyunsaturated oils with doses of omega-3 fatty acids) and extra virgin olive oil and peanut butter (monounsaturated oils).

Fish oils are best obtained through a consumption of salmon a minimum of three times a week. Fish oil caps are good, but you need at least 10 per day in order to get even 10 grams of fish oil.

Flax oil is best obtained from buying the whole ground flaxseed meal, which needs to be refrigerated at all times. I am fond of Bob's Red Mill Flaxseed Meal. Also available is the oil version, but researchers like Dr. Serrano have concluded that your best option is using meal rather than oil. If you choose to go with oil, the best brand to my knowledge is Spectrum. This company ensures the oil is refrigerated on the way from their manufacturing facilities to the nutrition stores. Do not cook with this oil as it is very light sensitive and heat sensitive. It should appear as a clear yellow. If you purchase oil with brown particles, the oil is rancid and should be returned or thrown out.

Extra virgin olive oil, a mono-unsaturated oil, should be preferably canned in Italy or Spain. It's best to purchase oil canned, because light can reach the oil stored in a bottle and make it rancid. Scott Mendelsohn, nutrition and training specialist and director of infinityfitness.com, pointed this out to me, and you will be amazed at the flavor difference in oils. Also, natural old-fashioned peanut butter is a great source of mono-unsaturated fats.

A product I feel needs to be mentioned is Serrano Labs' Alpha Omega M3. Developed by Dr. Eric Serrano, M.D., an expert in nutrition, these caps contain a combination of alpha linolenic acid, borage oil GLA, CLA (conjugated linolenic acid), EPA, DHA and vitamin E. They provide, in other words, almost all of the essential fats that your body needs, and I say almost all as the body still requires real fats from food. If you use 1 to 3 capsules taken with your mini-meals 1, 3, and 5, these can provide you with all of the good properties that good fats have to offer. What I truly like about these caps is the care taken during manufacturing to eliminate all the mercury typically found in poorly manufactured fish caps. If you choose to use these caps, I suggest that you do not count their grams of fats into your daily calculations. I've found the best prices for this product are at www.infinityfitness.com

To know how much of these fats to use and when, follow the recommendations in the nutrition chapter.

Vitamin C

Vitamin C is a water-soluble vitamin that improves your immune system and assists in faster recovery from your workouts. It suppresses the amount of cortisol (a hormone that kills muscle and aids in the accumulation of fat) released by your body during a workout. This is the only vitamin I recommend taking in megadose quantities. Because it is a water-soluble vitamin, it will not be stored by the body. If taken an hour before a workout (1000 mg dose), research shows vitamin C significantly reduces muscle soreness and speeds recovery.

I recommend a total of 3,000 mg per day of vitamin C. If your multiple-vitamin pack already has 1,000 mg, and you take this in the morning, then all you need is an extra 1,000 mg at lunch and 1,000 mg at dinner. For obtaining this, simply select a quality brand that sells tablets at a reasonable price. I personally use the ones sold at Sam's Club. Other good ones are the ones from the Vitamin Shoppe.

Chromium Picolinate

There are many claims surrounding chromium picolinate, and most of them are as yet unproven. However, I suggest its use from my own experience with this mineral. Some of its benefits include an enhanced effect on insulin, upgrading its capability to produce muscle and energy. An insulin-boosting vitamin could potentially assist in gaining muscle and losing fat faster. Chromium may also keep blood sugar levels stable, thereby preventing insulin levels from going high enough to begin promoting fat storage. However, chromium only functions if a suitable diet is followed.

Sources: All chromium picolinate produced in the market is manufactured by a company called Nutrition 21; it is sold at stores like GNC, Eckerds, Wal-Mart and Walgreens.

Quantity: 200 mcg with the post workout meal and with breakfast on days off.

Performance Enhancing Supplements (Highly Recommended for the Serious Trainer)

These supplements are suggested if you are both really serious about your training, and you can afford them.

Creatine Monohydrate

Creatine is a metabolite produced in the body composed of three amino acids: l-methionine, l-arginine, and l-glycine. Approximately 95% of the concentration is found in skeletal muscle in two forms: creatine phosphate and free chemically unbound creatine. The remaining 5% of the creatine stored in the body is found in the brain, heart and testes. The body of a sedentary person metabolizes and average of 2 grams of creatine a day. Bodybuilders due to their high intensity training metabolize higher amounts than that.

Creatine is generally found in red meats and to some extent in certain types of fish. However, it would be hard to get the amount of creatine necessary for performance enhancement as even though 2.2 lb of red meat or tuna contain approximately 4 to 5 grams of creatine, the compound is destroyed with cooking. Therefore, the best way to get creatine is by taking it in powder form.

How does it work?

While there is still much debate as to how creatine exerts its performance enhancing benefits, it is commonly accepted by now that most of its effects are due to two mechanisms:

- Intra-cellular water retention
- Creatine's ability to enhance ATP production

Basically, once the creatine is stored inside the muscle cell, it attracts the water surrounding the cell, thereby enlarging it. This super hydrated state of the cell causes nice side effects such as the increase of strength, and it also gives the appearance of a fuller muscle. Some studies suggest that a superhydrated cell may also trigger protein synthesis and minimize catabolism.

In addition, creatine provides for faster recovery in between sets and increased tolerance to high volume work. The way it does this is by enhancing the body's ability to produce adenosine triphosphate (ATP). ATP is the compound that your muscles use for fuel whenever they contract. ATP provides its energy by releasing one of its phosphate molecules (it has three phosphate molecules). After the release of the molecule, ATP becomes ADP (adenosine diphosphate) as it now only has two molecules. The problem is that after 10 seconds of contraction time the ATP fuel extinguishes and in order to support further muscle contraction glycolisis (glycogen burning) has to kick in. That is fine and well except for the fact that as a byproduct of that mechanism lactic acid is produced. Lactic acid is what causes the burning sensation at the end of the set. When too much lactic acid is produced, your muscle contractions stop, thereby forcing you to stop the set. However, by taking creatine, you can extend the 10 second limit of your ATP system as creatine provides ADP the phosphate molecule that it is missing (recall that creatine is stored in the muscle as creatine phosphate). By upgrading your body's ability of regenerating ATP, you can exercise longer and harder as you will minimize your lactic acid production and you will be able to take your sets to the next level and reduce fatigue levels. More volume, strength, and recovery equals more muscle (assuming nutrition and rest are dialed in).

Creatine also seems to allow for better pumps during a workout. This may be due to the fact that it possibly improves glycogen synthesis. In addition, studies have shown that creatine helps lower cholesterol and triglyceride levels. The mechanisms by which it exerts such benefits remain unknown.

In my own experimentation with creatine I have found that it provides all of the effects described above. As a way to prove to myself that these results were just not a placebo effect, I finally convinced my training partner (who was extremely skeptical about the compound) to start using it. After two weeks he noticed that for some reason he was recovering faster in between sets, and had a better tolerance to high volume work, and his muscles were looking fuller. He did not understand why that was happening. At that time I reminded him about the 5 grams of creatine that were being added to his post work-out protein shake. By the way, he has been body-building now for ten years so he is not a beginner. So while one subject does not provide me the statistical leverage to claim that creatine will provide these effects, I am positive that provided your training, rest, and nutrition are in order, you will get results.

Sources

Good brands of creatine are Prolab, Beverly International, EAS, Champion Nutrition, Labrada, Beverly International, Met-Rx and iSatori.

How to Use It

If you read the bottle, most companies recommend a loading phase of 20 grams for 5 days and 5 to 10 grams thereafter. While that is the commonly accepted way to use it, in my own experimentation I have found no benefit to loading. I have even gone as far as loading for 7 days with 40 grams a day and found no difference. As a matter of fact, my training partner only took 5 grams a day after the workout and started getting great results after only a couple of weeks. The reason for this is simple. There is only so much creatine that the body can store. Recall that the creatine is stored every time that you take it. So by taking it every day, eventually you will reach the upper levels that provideperformance enhancement. After you reach that level, you could get away with just taking it on your weight training days as it takes two weeks of no use for the body's creatine levels to get back to normal.

Since creatine is such a hot supplement, I decided to add some additional information on it at the end of this book. For more information on creatine, please refer to Appendix I.

Glutamine

L-Glutamine is the most abundant amino acid in muscle cells. It is released from the muscle during times of stress, such as hard weight training workouts and dieting. Not only proven to be an anti-catabolic agent that protects the muscle, it is also a contributor to muscle cell volume, and has immune system enhancing properties. It also helps in the following ways:

- Regulates protein synthesis
- Accelerates glycogen synthesis after a workout
- Spares the use of the glycogen stored in the muscle cell and directs use of other sources
- Speeds recuperation from weight training workouts

How to Use It

Due to its anti-catabolic properties and how it accelerates glycogen synthesis after a workout, glutamine is best taken 20 to 30 minutes after a workout with a protein shake. On days that you don't work out, take it with your last protein shake of the day. While there is much debate among experts as far as dosage is concerned, I suggest remaining on the conservative side, and believe 3 grams is a sufficient dosage. There is limited space within a muscle cell to store the glutamine, so taking higher dosages will not get you better results.

As far as cycling this supplement (or ceasing to use it for a set period of time) is concerned, there is no evidence that suggests cycling would improve its efficacy.

Side Effects

I used the straight powder form and experienced only a slight stomach discomfort during the first week of use. I did not experience any other side effects while using the compound and have not found any literature that links its use to any health problem. As normally advised, I recommend that you start with a low dosage (perhaps only 1 gram a day) to assess your tolerance. From there, you can easily build up to the recommended dosage of 3 grams.

Conclusion

After examining the results this supplement has been proven to give, as well as its easily accessible purchase price, I wonder why more athletes don't use it. Its benefits are especially important during dieting as a way to protect the muscle from being cannibalized. Remember that, as with any other supplement, you need to stick to high quality brands. Good brands of glutamine are available through Prolab, Beverly International, EAS, Champion Nutrition, Met-Rx, and Labrada.

Testosterone Boosting Supplements (Not Required but Worth Mentioning; Also Not to Be Used by Teenagers)

If you plan to compete, have the budget to try them, and are over 25, the age when your hormonal production has begun to decline, these are the supplements that you could take. Teenagers should stay away from any supplement that has an effect on their hormonal levels, as there is no need to upset a teen's delicate hormonal balance. Teenagers produce the equivalent of a 300 mg shot of testosterone per week; there is no need to increase the production of testosterone in a system already producing at peak levels.

The efficacy of some of these supplements is still under debate, but as a competitive athlete, I have seen an edge. I would like to mention that when you increase your hormonal levels, you could develop acne and a slightly increased aggression level. Finally, if you have the genetics for male pattern baldness, or an enlarged prostate, you should monitor these things if you decide to use these products. Blood work every 4 months is a wise investment if you choose to start manipulating hormone levels. Things to check for are liver enzymes, kidney function, PSA levels, cholesterol levels, thyroid levels, and any other test that your doctor may deem necessary.

ZMA

This scientifically-designed anabolic mineral formula consists of zinc monomethionine aspartate, magnesium aspartate and vitamin B-6. This all-natural product has been clinically proven to significantly increase anabolic hormone levels and muscle strength in trained athletes. Hard training athletes typically deplete the body of these essential minerals. Studies have shown that supplementing with 30 mg of zinc and 450 mg of magnesium per day can elevate testosterone levels up to 30%. I use Prolab's ZMA before bedtime.

TRIBULUS TERRESTRIS

This Bulgarian herb is believed to increase both free and total testosterone levels enhancing, as a result, your sex drive and muscle building capabilities. It is said to exert its effects by increasing luteninizing hormone (LH) levels, a hormone that signals the body to increase its testosterone production. This herb has been used for centuries for ailments such as headaches, premature ejaculation, water retention, and dizziness. Some research indicates that it has properties that assist in protection of the liver and the cardiovascular system as well. This herb is produced in a product by Biotest labs named Tribex 500. This product also contains a very useful herb called avena sativa.

AVENA SATIVA

Avena sativa, better known as wild oat, is an annual grass cultivated for its edible grain. It has the effect of increasing free testosterone levels, the testosterone that can be used by the body. While how this functions is not yet clear, it is suspected that it increases LH levels, similar to tribulus. Because these two supplements seem to work together, Biotest Labs included both herbs in their product Tribex 500. I take 3 capsules twice a day on an empty stomach only from Monday through Friday.

RED-KAT

Another product produced by Biotest Laboratories, Red-Kat is a hormone-free formula designed to increase the free testosterone levels in males. The two main ingredients in the formula are Eurycoma longifolia jack and Sclaremax. Eurycoma longifolia Jack, commonly known as tongkat in Malaysia, is a plant reputed to have aphrodisiac properties. Sclaremax's effects include antithrombotics and antidepressants, as well as stimulating the luteinizing hormone, resulting in the production of testosterone in males. I use 2 capsules with my Tribex 500 (twice a day) from Monday through Friday.

6-OXO

6-OXO, short for 3,6,17-androstenetrione, increases testosterone levels naturally by suppressing estrogen levels. Males produce this hormone largely when the aromatase enzyme converts testosterone into estrogen. 6-OXO binds to the aromatase enzyme and renders it ineffective, which increases testosterone levels. I take 3 capsules of 6-OXO with my ZMA at night with my last meal. The product I use is made by ErgoPharm.

Other Supplements (Not Recommended)

This section is dedicated to the supplements that many questions are asked about. Some of these may soon be banned by the government, so discussion is limited to the very basics.

NO2

Nitric oxide, a free-form gas, is produced in the body and used for cell-to-cell communication. Enzymes in the body break down the amino acid Arginine to produce NO^2.

Nitric oxide increases blood flow to the muscle, which makes it interesting to bodybuilders, as increased blood flow may serve to deliver additional nutrients to muscles, helping muscles to become larger when subjected to stress.

However, I have seen no research to indicate that taking a supplement keeps your nitric oxide levels elevated. There is research that links chronically elevated levels of NO^2 to immune disorders and increased inflammation. I have never tried this supplement myself, and those who have claim to see benefits, and report that a large pump was experienced but that it disappeared after cessation of use. In my opinion the product is too expensive for what it claims to do, and it may soon be linked to immune disorders.

ANDROSTENDIONE

The government is in the process of banning these hormones, but many questions are raised about them. I'll discuss what androstendione and pro hormones really are and why you should stay away from most of them.

Producers of androstenedione, the most popular pro hormone, and other pro hormone supplements, claim their products increase testosterone levels to a level otherwise unobtainable. These claims assume that the body will convert all of the ingested androstendione into testosterone, which is incorrect. While a portion of the androstenedione ingested may be turned into testosterone, there is a possibility, depending on your body, that it may instead be turned into estrogen. Also, please remember that when you introduce a foreign hormone into the body, the body shuts down the natural production of that hormone to keep it balanced. By ingesting androstenedione, you may be stopping your natural testosterone production. Some studies also suggest that Androstenedione creates side effects like increased acne, aggressiveness, and a higher chance of baldness.

Not only does this compound not work, but it also brings risks if you use it. Since pro hormones are technically steroids, they have many of the same problems, but not the success rate of the prescription-only versions. A study recently published in the Journal of the American Medical Association examined the short and long-term effects of androstenedione. In the short-term study, 10 of 30 men received a one-time dose of 100 mg of androstenedione. In the long-term study, the remaining 20 performed 8 weeks of resistance training and received either 300 mg of androstenedione or a placebo daily. The androstenedione/resistance training groups did not

experience a rise in any form of testosterone, or an increase in strength. However, they did experience a rise in LDL (low-density lipoprotein) cholesterol, commonly known as bad cholesterol, and a rise in estrogen. My question to you is this: Would you take a supplement with almost identical side effects to steroids, without receiving any of the benefits steroids do offer?

1-AD *and* 1-TEST

In an effort to eliminate the issues of androstenedione, more pro hormones were developed. The two most powerful are named 1-AD and 1-Test. Having said that, these pro hormones do not increase estrogen levels and do work at relatively low levels (around 300 mg). The downside is there will be an increase in your aggression, and your natural testosterone production will plummet with your sex drive. These supplements may also accelerate hair loss and enlarge your prostate. They will not kill you, but these are definitely not harmless substances.

These compounds were just made illegal on October 22, 2004, by President Bush as he signed the 2004 Steroid Control Act. Therefore, possession of these items will land you 5 years in prison. Therefore, the discussion presented here was merely for educational purposes.

I prefer to increase my testosterone levels through smart training, nutrition, rest, and safe supplements.

Steroids; The Bad, the Good, and the Ugly

Steroids are not a nutritional supplement, but I felt compelled to touch on this subject.

The purpose of this section is not to teach you how to use steroids, nor to endorse or disapprove of their use. This is an informational tool to answer questions on the subject, as well as to eliminate misconceptions that surround these drugs. Everything that I have said is based on research and information gathered from others that have used them. I cannot share any personal experiences as I have never touched them.

WHAT ARE THEY?

Anabolic steroids are a synthetic copy of the hormone testosterone. Athletes, especially bodybuilders, may feel lured towards them as these drugs do increase muscle size, strength, and stamina. One of the biggest myths about steroids is that if you take them they will kill you. Steroids are drugs. All drugs when misused or abused have the potential to kill.

Another myth is that they are easily accessible, and there is only one type of steroid. Unless you get steriods prescribed by a doctor, steroids are illegal substances and only available through the black market, and their quality is largely a mystery. If you are caught with them in your possession without a prescription you can face up to 5 years in a federal prison. There are many different types of steroids out there. There are liquid steroids (injectables) and there are pills. Liquid steroids are more anabolic and less dam-

aging to organs like the liver. The oral versions are more androgenic and have more side effects than injectables. Some steroids build muscle mass, while others increase strength or decrease fat. As properties vary, so do their side effects. The stronger the steroid, especially if orally administered, the more drastic the side effects.

THE GOOD

Steroids do increase size and strength, and they do so very significantly. In addition to gains in strength and muscle mass, they also appear to provide you with energy and aggressiveness, both very conducive to good workouts. Depending on the steroid, you may also experience cell voluminizing effects that create a bigger pump. These benefits assume that all aspects of the bodybuilding program (training, nutrition, and supplementation) are working.

THE BAD

It should come as no surprise that steroids create a psychological dependence. After approximately 8 weeks of use, steroid users have an "unstoppable" feeling. Once you stop using them, you likely will notice that your pumps are down, your strength is diminishing, and your muscle mass is shrinking. Also, for the first few weeks off of the steroids, bouts of depression are likely due to your low testosterone levels.

Add all of this up, and it is no wonder that a large number of steroid users never stop taking these drugs.

THE UGLY

Assuming you began steroid use with all the precautions (consistent blood work taken, using a mild steroid, double checking the dosage amount, tapering off before stopping use, and not using every 12 weeks or so), chances are high that you will still experience depression, loss of strength, and loss of muscle mass. You will also likely notice a period of low natural testosterone production in addition to side effects encountered during their use, such as higher blood pressure and higher cholesterol levels. I have seen research claiming that the administration of mild steroids can aid in maintaining a percentage of the muscle mass gains. This is, however, dependent on many variables: the type of steroids used, their quantity, and the anti-estrogen drugs taken after going off the drugs. Most do not have the information on how to go about this unless the steroids are prescribed by a doctor, and as a result, I have never heard of a steroid user keeping his gains after steroid use ended. For most people, steroid use will ultimately provide many more losses than it will provide gains.

If you are careless with your steroid use and possibly use high potency steroids or abuse the dosage administered, then the side effects will be numerous during the period of use, and you also will experience terrible side effects once use has ended. The degree of side effects you experience is dependant on the dosage and type of the steroid, as well as your genetic propensity. It's impossible to precisely predict what type and how many side effects a user will encounter during steroid use. However, below is a list of a few of the known side effects of steroid abuse:

- Increased liver function
- Compromised testosterone levels
- Increase in cholesterol levels and blood pressure
- Altered thyroid function
- Migraine headaches
- Nose bleeds
- Muscle cramps
- Development of breast-like tissue in men (Gynecomastia AKA "bitch tits")
- Insulin insensitivity
- Androgenic side effects such as thinning hair, enlarged prostate, oily skin, water retention, increased body hair, and physical aggressiveness
- Stunted growth, if taken while in your teen years
- Possible acceleration in the growth of tumors.
- In addition to the above, the oral steroids also cause nausea, diarrhea, constipation, and vomiting

I'm not even going to discuss the kind of disastrous side effects that occur when females decide to use steroids. They are in essence administering the opposite sex hormones to their body!

For a better idea of what each particular steroid does, please visit the following link at Mesomorphosis.com: http://www.mesomorphosis.com/steroid-profiles/index.htm

Supplement Recommendations Summary

Essential To Take

- Multivitamin/mineral complex taken with breakfast

- Essential oils and monounsaturated oils as per nutrition section

- 1 gram vitamin C taken with breakfast, lunch, and dinner

- Whey gain, whey protein powder, or meal replacement powder to mix with skim milk or water to make protein shakes

- 200mcg of Chromium Picolinate taken with protein shake after the workout

- 3-4 Beverly International's Ultra 40 Beef Liver Tablets with each meal.

Highly Recommended

(Only useful if you are really pushing your workouts to the limit)

- 2.5 grams of creatine before and after the workout

- 3 grams of glutamine after the workout or before bed on non-workout days

For trainees over 25 years old who wish to increase their testosterone levels

- ZMA (1 serving with evening meal)

- Tribex 500 (3 capsules twice daily—A.M./P.M.—on empty stomach from Mon to Fri)

- Red Kat (2 capsules twice daily-A.M./P.M.-on empty stomach from Mon to Fri)

- 6-OXO (3 capsules at night every day)

There is no need to take all of these supplements at the same time. You could get great benefit from doing 6 weeks of one, 6 weeks of another and so on. However, if you have the finances to use them all there is no adverse effect from doing so.

NOTE: Just recently a new supplement made by Sylvester Stallone's new nutrition company called InStone, came into the market. It combines the ZMA, the Tribulus and the 6-OXO all in one product. The product is called Forza-T and retails for $43.95 at the moment at www.body-building.com. It contains 20 servings. Not bad considering that it has all of these supplements in one product.

Conclusion

I am not going say: "Don't use steroids; they kill." By now you can make an educated conclusion yourself. Many drugs are available over-the-counter and by prescription that in my opinion are far more dangerous than steroids. I do feel that steroids have their place in medicine for those that do not produce adequate levels of testosterone. If this is the case for you, a doctor can determine if replacement therapy is in order.

However, it seems to me that using steroids with a perfectly functioning hormonal system only provides fleeting glory and is only a temporary solution for acquiring muscle mass. You might get bigger in the short term, but how much is that worth? Is it worth risking your health and going to jail? If you purchase the drugs on the black market, how can you be assured of their quality? Will they contain contaminants? If you are using an injectable steroid, will you be able to consistently inject it correctly? How can you be sure you are not on the path to developing cancer and, by using steroids, assisting in its growth? All of these things you should consider if tempted to buy these drugs from someone other than a medical professional. Building your body into a beautiful work of art should start with a lifetime commitment. There are no shortcuts to its hard work; not even steroids function without hard work. Relatively hard work combined with smart training and a sound nutrition system will take you exactly where you want to go.

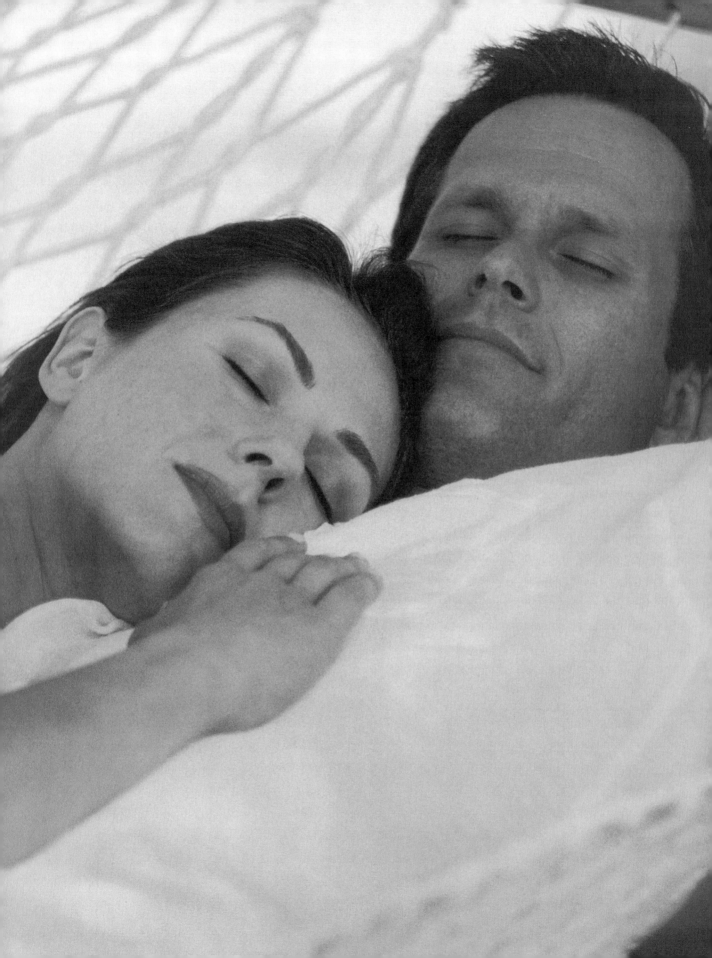

CHAPTER 6

Rest and Recovery

Rest and recovery is the most neglected component in a bodybuilding program. If you neglect this, get ready for a lifetime of no gains. In order to grow the body has to recover, and that happens when we sleep.

The Sleep Cycle

When we deprive ourselves of sleep, we disrupt a very delicate cycle.

Phase One: Phase one starts when the sun sets and the pineal gland begins to release melatonin, the hormone responsible for sleepiness which is released in the absence of light. When you lie down at this time, muscles relax, heart rate and breathing slow down, and body temperature drops. The brain also relaxes but still remains alert. If you could look at the brain's wave patterns, you would see a change from the rapid beta waves of daytime to slower alpha waves. When the alpha waves disappear, replaced by theta waves, the sleeper has tumbled into stage one sleep. In this stage, the sleeper is unable to sense anything.

Phase Two: Phase two occurs moments after phase one, and in this stage the sleeper lies still for 10 to 15 minutes.

Phase Three: After phase two, the sleeper falls into a deeper sleep, generally lasting 5 to 15 minutes.

Phase Four: Once a maximum of 15 minutes are spent in phase three, the sleeper falls into the relaxed stage called phase four, lasting a half hour or so. In stage four, the eyes move back and forth very quickly in what is named rapid eye movement (REM). This is when the first dream occurs. Once it ends, the sleeper returns to phase two and restarts the process.

These processes repeat themselves about five times during the night.

Studies tell us the average person sleeps approximately 8 hours and fifteen minutes when uninterrupted. During these studies, there were no alarm clocks or disturbing noises to interrupt normal sleep patterns. Eight hours and fifteen minutes is believed to be the ideal physiological time the body requires for sleep.

Maladies Caused By Sleep Deprivation

These are the maladies that, according to research, could result from consistent sleep deprivation:

Impaired glucose tolerance. Without sleep, the central nervous system increases activity, which blocks the pancreas from producing adequate insulin, the hormone the body requires to digest glucose. Researcher Van Cauten, who conducted a study on sleep deprivation on healthy young men with no risk factors, said, "In one week, we had them in a pre-diabetic state."

Possible link to obesity. During the first round of deep sleep, much of the body's growth hormone is secreted. As both men and women age, they naturally spend less time in deep sleep, which reduces the growth hormone present in the body. Lack of sleep at a younger age, however, lowers growth hormone prematurely, and accelerates as a result the fat-gaining process. There is also research indicating a lowered testosterone level as well, which would make fat gain and muscle loss an easy thing.

Increased carbohydrate cravings. Sleep depravation negatively affects the production of a hormone called leptin, the hormone responsible for telling the body when it is full. With a decreased production, your body craves calories (especially in the form of carbs) even after its requirements are met.

Weakened immune system. Research indicates sleep deprivation adversely affects white blood cell counts and the body's ability to fight infections.

Increased levels of estrogen. Richard Stevens, a cancer researcher at the University of Connecticut Health Center, speculated there might be a connection between breast cancer and hormone cycles disrupted by late-night light. Melatonin, primarily secreted at night, may trigger a reduction in the body's production of estrogen. Light interferes with melatonin release, which is only secreted in response to a lack of light, and allows estrogen levels to rise. Too much estrogen is known to promote the growth of breast cancer even in men.

Decreased alertness and ability to focus. A recent study showed that those awake for up to 19 hours scored worse on performance tests and alertness scales than those with a blood-alcohol level of .08 percent (legally drunk in some states).

Hardening of the arteries. Some studies suggest that stress imposed on the body due to its lack of sleep causes a very sharp rise in cortisol levels. This imbalance could lead to hardening of the arteries, and then to a heart attack. Very high cortisol levels lead to muscle loss, increased fat storage, loss of bone mass, depression, hypertension, insulin resistance (cells in the body lose the ability to accept insulin), lower growth hormone, and lower testosterone production.

Depression and irritability. Lack of sleep causes the depletion of neurotransmitters in the brain in charge of regulating moods. Because of this, sleep deprived people have a "short fuse" and can get depressed easily.

Are You Sleep Deprived?

If you can lie down in the middle of the day and fall asleep within 10 minutes, you are sleep deprived. Catching up is basic math. For every minute under eight hours, you need an equal extra amount of time asleep soon after. If you're hundreds of hours in debt, you may never pay it all off. According to recent research, 17 hours was all the catching up people could do, and it generally took three weeks. Most people probably need three times that amount of sleep!

Sleeping Pills

Beware of sleeping pills! They not only tend to be addicting but people that use them tend to wake up groggy. Scientists are also divided in opinions when discussing melatonin supplementation, but most agree that the 3-milligram dose widely available is far too high, especially because it has never been tested safely in humans. I suggest that, instead of depending on chemicals, you follow the guidelines below for a good night's sleep:

Avoid activities that involve deep concentration. These activities will increase adrenaline levels and will prevent the brain from achieving the state of relaxation required to achieve sleep.

Avoid watching disturbing shows at night on TV. This may also increase your adrenaline levels, preventing you from a good night's sleep.

Avoid eating a large meal at night. Your digestion process will prevent you from falling asleep.

Attempt to totally relax at the same time each night. If you follow this rule, you condition your body to relax itself at the same time every day. At this time no thoughts other than those about relaxation and falling asleep should come to your head. You will need to learn how to block thoughts concerning work or other life issues. Listening to soothing music set at a low volume with the lights off can help you relax and achieve the state necessary to go to sleep.

Training While You Are Sick

Besides injuries, nothing has the ability to stall progress more than colds. If you are trying to decide if you should train or not, ask yourself: Am I suffering from a cold or the flu? Many people confuse the common cold with the flu, but these are different types of illnesses. The flu is caused by viruses known as Influenza A or Influenza B while the common cold is caused by viruses called coronaviruses and rhinoviruses. There are over 200 different types of these coronaviruses and rhinoviruses, and once you are hit, your immune system builds a lifelong immunity to that specific virus.

The flu is much more severe as usually accompanied by an array of body aches and fever. Your body's immune system is taxed much more severely by the flu than by the common cold. If you are suffering from the flu, training would be detrimental to your muscle growth and to your health as well. While training helps us gain muscle, lose fat, feel good, and become energetic, it is a catabolic activity, and the body needs to be in good health to gain the benefits of exercise. If you have the flu, weight training would only negatively affect the immune system fighting the virus. Do not train if you have the flu! Instead, concentrate on very good nutrition and drink large amounts of fluids (water and electrolyte replacement drinks like Propel and Pedialyte are an excellent option to prevent dehydration). Once the flu is gone, you can slowly start up your weight-training program with light weights (use the active recovery routine for 2 weeks or so). Do not push yourself too hard during the first week. During the second week, again use the active recovery routine but push yourself closer to muscular failure, still saving those last few reps. By the third week you should be back on track, so you can either repeat the active recovery routine but reach muscle failure, or return to the beginning of the phase where you left off.

If you have the common cold and the particular virus is mild (possibly just a runny nose and some coughing), you can train as long as you stop the sets short of reaching failure and decrease the weights by 25% in order to prevent too hard a push. However, if the cold virus hitting you makes you feel run down and achy, and comes with a sore throat and headaches, it would be best to stop training all together until the symptoms subside. If this is the case, follow the exercise program startup recommendations for after the flu. We do not want to make it any harder for the immune system to fight off a virus.

Always consult your doctor if you don't recognize your illness. Unfortunately, for most sicknesses, you will need to stop training and follow the advice given for training after the flu.

The flu and colds can throw a wrench on progress, so let's see how we can prevent these from affecting us.

Flu and Cold Prevention

Attacking generally during the winter months, flus and colds still must enter your system to affect you. It's best to implement a twofold prevention approach:

Prevent the virus from infiltrating your system. Cold viruses are spread by human contact. They get into your system through your mouth, eyes, and nose, and they can remain active for up to three hours. To assist in preventing them from taking root you can:

- Keep your hands away from your face
- Wash your hands with anti-bacterial soap frequently throughout the day, and always when you finish your workout at the gym

Maintain immune system operation at peak efficiency levels at all times. Exercise, a bad diet, and losing sleep all result in catabolic rebuilding. You can help prevent the bad effects by:

• Avoiding overtraining

• Maintaining a balanced diet, and avoiding processed foods with high levels of saturated fats, refined flours, or sugar

• Getting a healthy dose of sleep a day (anywhere from 7 to 9 hours depending on your individual requirements)

Stay healthy by following these tips and if you get sick, then rest until you get better. If you don't, you will end up more seriously ill and this will keep you out of the gym for a longer period of time than if you had rested.

Soreness

There are several degrees of soreness that we need to be aware of:

• Delayed onset muscle soreness

• Typical mild muscle soreness

• Injury-type muscle soreness

The first type of soreness is delayed onset muscle soreness (DOMS). The term DOMS refers to the deep muscular soreness usually experienced 2 days (not 1 day) after the exercise has been done. This prevents the full muscular contraction of that muscle. When you begin to train harder than you have before, this is the severe soreness that appears as a result. The pain could last between a couple of days for an advanced well-conditioned athlete, to as much as a week for someone just beginning. If you are affected by this soreness and it is time to work out again, I find that the best plan is to exercise

the body part following an active recovery routine where you still perform your prescribed routine, but all of the loads are reduced by 50% and the sets are not taken to muscular failure. You should also stop exercising once you reach repetition ten, well before you hit muscle failure. This workout should restore full movement in the muscle and remove lactic acid and other waste. Also, forcing high concentrations of blood into the damaged area will bring nutrients needed for repair and growth. This will work the muscle, and the next day it will not be as sore or stiff.

The second type of soreness is the typical mild muscle soreness experienced the day after a good workout. This soreness is more of a tenderness or slight burn in the trained muscle, unlike the sharp debilitating pain of DOMS. It is informally accepted that this burn is caused by micro-trauma at the muscle fiber level and an excess of lactic acid. This is good soreness; it is mild and muscle function is not impaired. It generally lasts a day or two for advanced athletes and can reach three days for a beginner. When you no longer experience this type of soreness the day after a workout it is an indication that your body has successfully adapted to the training program and you will see no gains unless the routine is changed.

The third type of soreness is caused by injury. Entirely different in nature from the ones described above, it usually is immobilizing in nature and accompanied by very sharp pains. Depending on its nature, it may only be experienced when the muscle is moved in a certain way

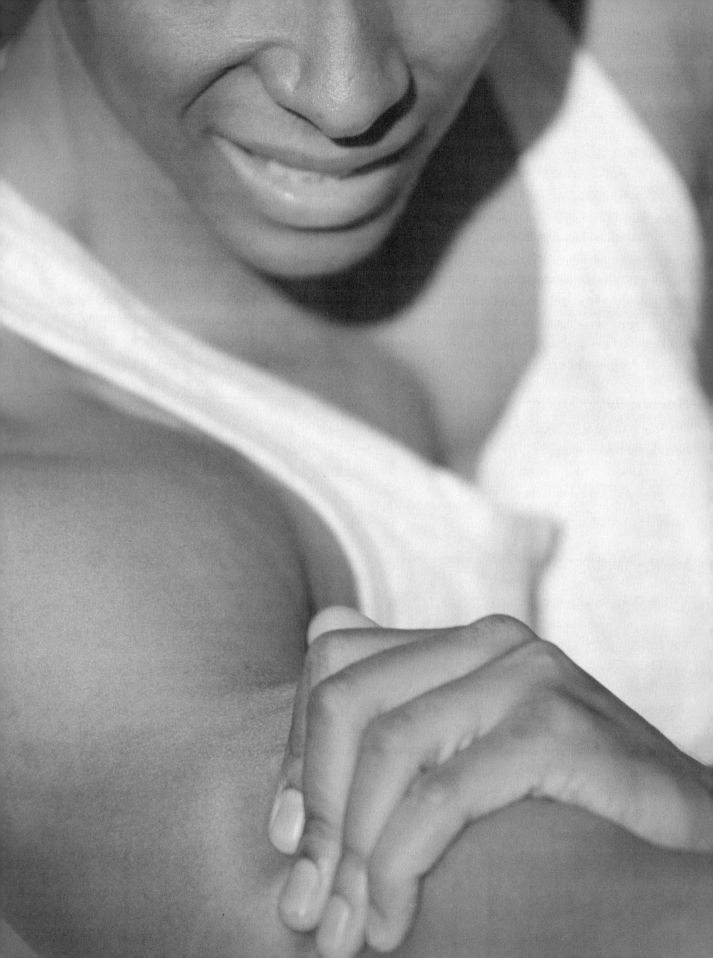

or repetitively. On occasion, these injuries are apparent immediately, and other times the day after. If you are injured, you should apply the RICE principle immediately (Recovery, Ice, Compression, and Elevation).

Should you consult a doctor? Some injuries allow you to continue training by working around the injury, or finding exercises that target the injured muscle without involving the range of motion that triggers pain. More serious injuries, like a muscle tear, could involve the complete rest of the injured area and even surgery.

When you weight train, please leave the ego behind. If it enters the weight room it could cause injuries that take you out of the gym, and return to haunt you long after the recovery period. The best way to prevent soreness is to cycle your exercise parameters and always practicing good form.

Overtraining

Overtraining is a condition caused when the body is taxed beyond its ability to recover. The causes include long workouts, high volume (too many sets and reps), and a bad diet. People who are overtrained lose muscle mass, feel weak, have trouble sleeping, lose appetite, feel lethargic and tired, and may become depressed.

This system should make it impossible for you to overtrain (assuming that you follow the nutrition and the rest recommendations) because the workouts are limited to 1 hour and are cycled adequately, and training occurs in 2 day blocks and leaves the weekends for rest. This program also enforces an active recovery period ever 6

weeks for the nervous system to recover from the heavy lifting. The nutrients provided by the diet, and the recommended supplements and rest schedule, also eliminate the possibility of overtraining.

I have heard claims that the training volume for hardgainers should be greatly reduced, and I disagree with this. If hardgainers have a nutrition plan, a lifestyle free of drug use, and adequate sleep, hardgainers are able to train at a much higher level than some think.

For the purposes of this book, overtraining is a state of mind and does not exist.

Conclusion

In conclusion, you need 7 to 9 hours of sleep (8 1/4 being the ideal) each night for your body to run efficiently. Deprive your body of sleep and you'll have lousy fat loss. You will also have muscle loss, which lowers your metabolism. You will lack energy and focus to work out. It will also lead to overtraining, as your recovery process stalls. There is also research that indicates that lack of sleep causes cravings and hardening of the arteries, potentially leading to a heart attack. If you don't think that you have enough time to sleep, then turn off the TV and make the time!

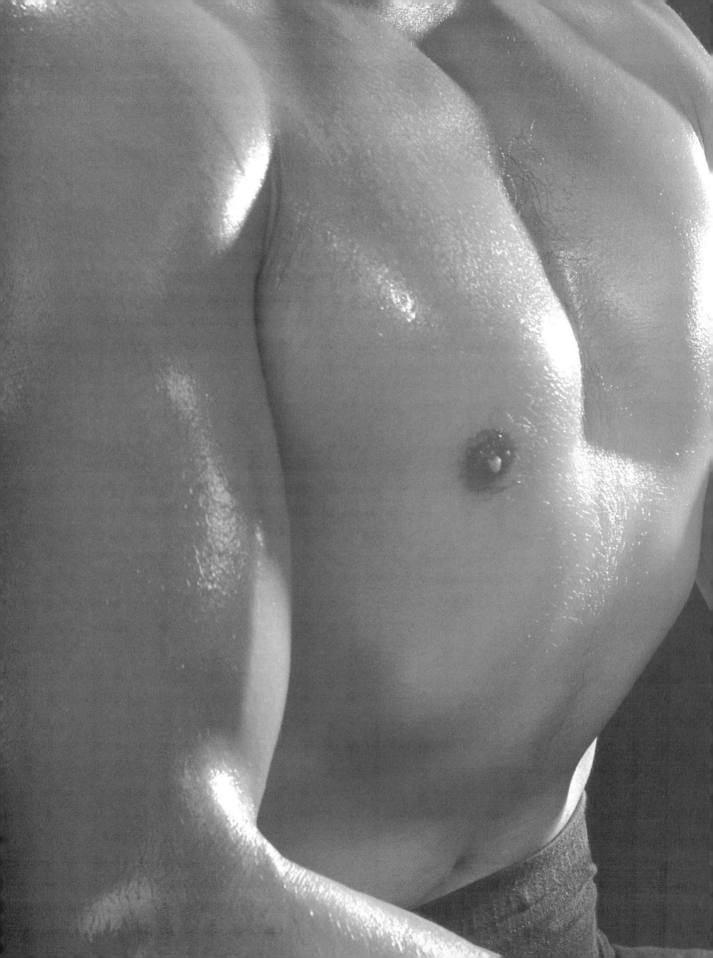

CHAPTER 7

Chest Exercises

BASIC EXERCISES

Incline Dumbbell Press

Dumbbell Bench Press

Incline Barbell Press

Chest Dips

ISOLATION EXERCISES

Cable Incline Flies

Dumbbell Pullovers

ALTERNATIVE EXERCISES

Barbell Bench Press (Basic)

Push-Ups (Basic)

Incline Bench Flies (Isolation)

Flat Bench Flies (Isolation)

Standing Cable Crossovers (Isolation)

The chest is a muscle that consists of two parts, the upper and lower regions. In order to have the appearance of a full chest, the size of both parts needs to be in proportion. An emphasis should be placed upon the upper part, as this gives the illusion of a larger chest. The upper chest also responds more slowly to exercise than the lower.

We will now cover the exercises used in this program, and at the end of the chapter, some additional useful exercises that can be used in lieu of the recommended ones are also included.

Incline Dumbbell Press

1 Lie back on an incline bench with a dumbbell in each hand resting on your thighs. The palms of your hand should face each other.

2 To get to the starting position, using your thighs to help you get the dumbbells up, clean the dumbbells one arm at a time to better hold them apart at shoulder width. Then rotate your wrists forward until the palms of your hands face away from you.

3 Lower the weights slowly to your sides as you inhale. Control the dumbbells at all times.

4 As you exhale, use your pectoral muscles to push the dumbbells up. Lock your arms in this contracted position, hold for a measured second and then start lowering the weights slowly. It should take at least twice as long to go down as to come up.

5 Repeat steps 3 and 4 for the pre-agreed amount of repetitions.

6 When finished, place the dumbbells back on your thighs and then on the floor. This is the safest way to set the dumbbells down.

Variations: If your incline bench is adjustable, you can use several angles. One variation has the palms of the hands facing each other. Another variation requires you to perform the exercise with palms facing each other, and twisting the wrists during the lift, so that at the top of the movement the palms are facing away from the body. I personally do not use this variation very often, as it seems to be hard on my shoulders.

Incline Dumbbell Press

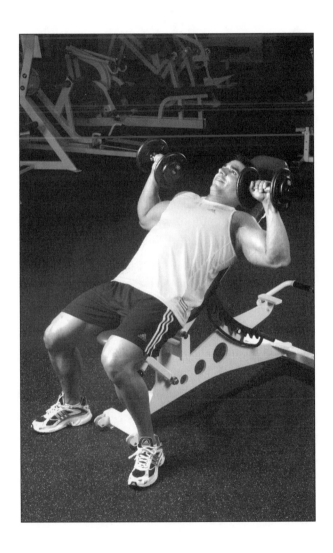
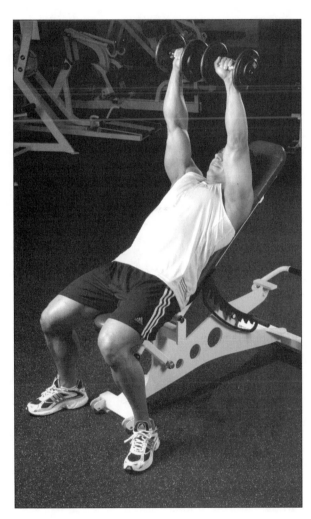

Dumbbell Bench Press

1 Lie down on a flat bench with a dumbbell in each hand resting on your thighs. The palms of your hand should face each other.

2 To move into the starting position, use your thighs to help you get the dumbbells up. Clean the dumbbells one arm at a time so they are held in front of you at shoulder width. Then rotate your wrists forward until the palms of your hands face away from you.

3 Lower the weights slowly to your side as you inhale. Control the dumbbells at all times.

4 As you exhale, use your pectoral muscles to push the dumbbells up. Lock your arms in the contracted position, hold for a measured second and then start lowering the dumbbells slowly. It should take at least twice as long to go down as to come up.

5 Repeat steps 3 and 4 for the pre-agreed amount of repetitions.

6 When you are finished, do not drop the dumbbells next to you. This is dangerous to the rotator cuff in your shoulders, as well as to others working out around you. Just lift your legs from the floor, bending at your knees, and twist your wrists so the palms of your hands face each other. Place the dumbbells on top of your thighs. When both dumbbells are touching your thighs simultaneously, push your upper torso up while pressing the dumbbells on your thighs, and kick slightly forward with your legs. Make sure to keep the dumbbells on top of the thighs. This momentum will help you get back to a sitting position with both dumbbells still on top of your thighs, at which point you can place the dumbbells on the floor safely.

Variations: Another variation of this exercise is to perform it with the palms of the hands facing each other. This variation is good for the second time you go through this program. Also, you can perform the exercise with the palms facing each other and then twisting the wrist as you lift the dumbbells so that at the top of the movement the palms are facing away from the body. I personally do not use this variation very often, as it seems to be hard on my shoulders.

Dumbbell Bench Press

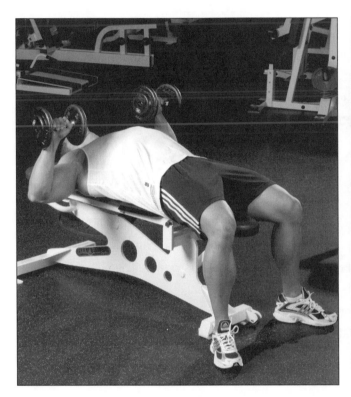 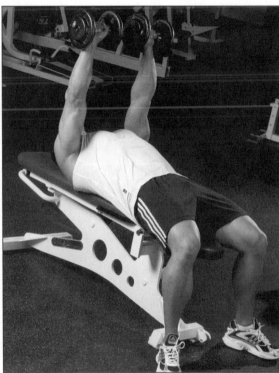

Incline Barbell Press

① Lie back on an incline bench. Using a medium width grip (a grip that creates a 90-degree angle in the middle of the movement between the forearms and the upper arms), lift the bar from the rack and hold it straight over you with your arms locked. This will be your starting position.

② As you breathe in, come down slowly until you feel the bar on you upper chest.

③ After a second pause, bring the bar back to the starting position as you breathe out and push the bar using your chest muscles. Lock your arms in the contracted position, hold for a second and then start coming down slowly again (it should take at least twice as long to go down as to come up).

④ Repeat the movement for the prescribed amount of repetitions.

⑤ When you are done, place the bar back in the rack.

Caution: If you are new at this exercise, it is advised that you use a spotter. If no spotter is available, then be conservative with the amount of weight used. Also, beware of letting the bar drift too far forward. You want the bar to fall on your upper chest and nowhere else.

Variations: You can use several angles on the incline bench if the one you are using is adjustable.

Incline Barbell Press

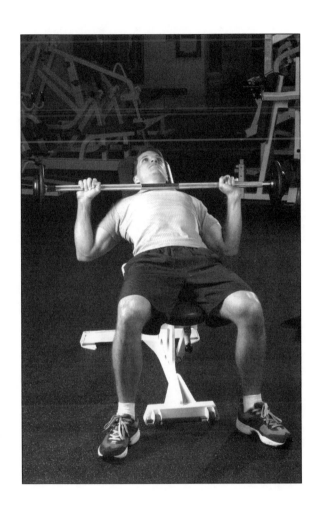 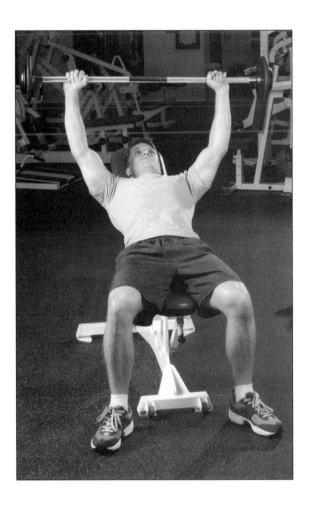

Chest Dips

1 For this exercise you will need access to parallel bars. To get yourself into the starting position, hold your body at arm's length (arms locked) above the bars.

2 While breathing in, lower yourself slowly with your torso leaning forward around 30 degrees or so and your elbows flared out slightly until you feel a slight stretch in the chest.

3 Once you feel the stretch, use your chest to bring your body back to the starting position as you breathe out.

4 Repeat the movement for the prescribed amount of repetitions.

Variations: If you are new at this exercise and do not have the strength to perform it, use a dip assist machine if available. These machines use weight to help you push your body weight. Otherwise, a spotter holding your legs can help. If none of these two options are available, then substitute a barbell bench press, which is described later in this chapter. On the other hand, more advanced lifters can add weight to the exercise by using a weight belt that allows the addition of weighted plates.

Chest Dips

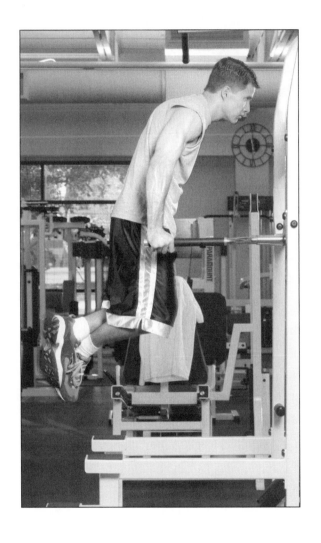 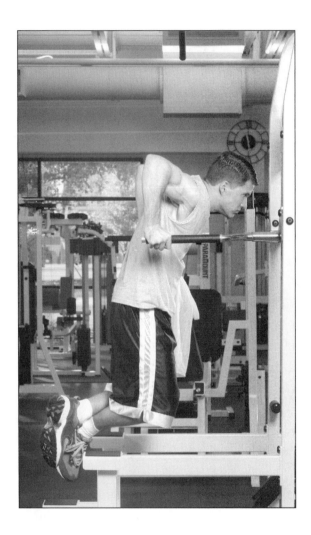

Cable Incline Flies

1 For this exercise you will need access to a pulley machine. To get yourself into the starting position, set the pulleys at the floor level (lowest level possible on the machine that is below your torso), place an incline bench (set at 45 degrees) in between the pulleys, select a weight on each one and grab a pulley on each hand.

2 With a handle on each hand, lie on the incline bench and bring your hands together at arms length in front of your face.

3 With a slight bend on your elbows in order to prevent stress at the biceps tendon, lower your arms out at both sides in a wide arc until you feel a stretch on your chest. Breathe in as you perform this portion of the movement. Keep in mind that throughout the movement, the arms should remain stationary; the movement should only occur at the shoulder joint.

4 Return your arms back to the starting position as you breathe out. Make sure to use the same arc of motion used to lower the weights.

5 Hold for a second at the starting position and repeat the movement for the prescribed amount of repetitions.

Variations: You can vary the angle of the bench in order to target the upper chest at slightly different angles.

Notes: For the incline flies, use the low pulleys of the cable machine to make sure that you get a nice stretch at the bottom and a nice contraction at the top.

Cable Incline Flies

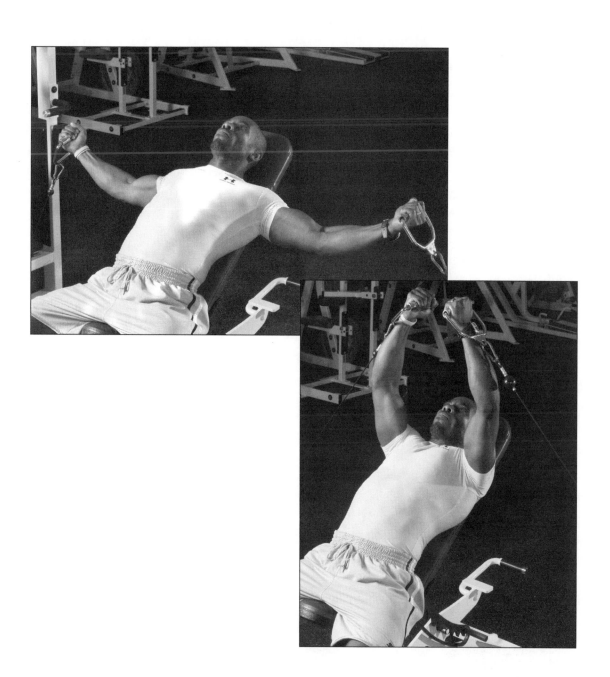

Dumbbell Pullovers

① Place a dumbbell standing up on a flat bench.

② Ensuring that the dumbbell stays securely placed at the top of the bench, lie perpendicular to the bench (torso across it as if forming a cross) with only your shoulders lying on the surface. Hips should be below the bench and legs bent with feet firmly on the floor. The head will be off the bench as well.

③ Grasp the dumbbell with both hands and hold it straight over your chest at arm's length. Both palms should be pressing against the underside of one of the ends of the dumbbell. This will be your starting position.

④ While keeping your arms straight, lower the weight slowly in an arc behind your head while breathing in until you feel a stretch on both the chest and the lats.

⑤ At that point, bring the dumbbell back to the starting position using the arc through which the weight was lowered and exhale as you perform this movement.

⑥ Hold the weight on the initial position for a second and repeat the motion for the prescribed number of repetitions.

Caution: If you are new to this movement, have a spotter hand you the weight instead. If not, please ensure that the dumbbell does not fall on you as you arrange your torso to perform the exercise on the bench. Also, ensure that the dumbbell used is in perfect working condition. Old dumbbells in need of welding should never be used to perform this exercise.

Variations: You can perform this exercise using a barbell or an E-Z bar instead of dumbbells. Also, if using dumbbells like Powerblocks, just use a dumbbell on each hand with the palms of your hands facing each other.

Dumbbell Pullovers

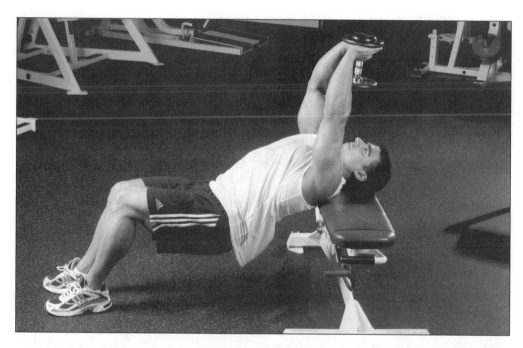

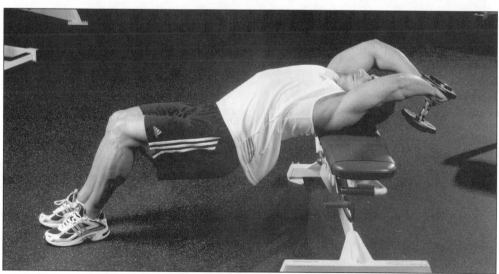

Barbell Bench Press

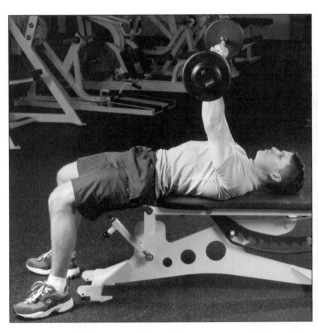
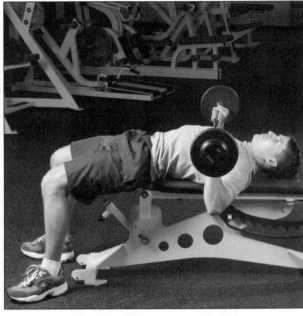

❶ Lie back on a flat bench. To enter the starting position, lift the bar from the rack and hold it straight over you with your arms locked, your hands in a medium width grip.

❷ As you inhale, lower the bar slowly until you can feel the bar on your middle chest.

❸ Pause, then return the bar to the starting position by exhaling and pushing the bar using your chest muscles. Lock your arms in the contracted position, hold for a second and then come down slowly, taking at least twice as long to go down as to come up.

❹ When you are done, place the bar back in the rack.

Caution: You should have a spotter. If not, then be conservative with how much weight you use. Also beware of letting the bar drift too far forward; it should fall on your middle chest and nowhere else.

Push-Ups

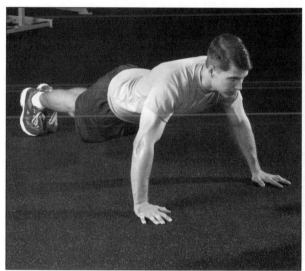 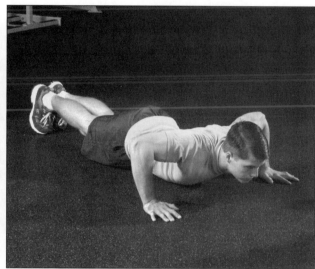

1 Lie on the floor face down and place your hands about 36 inches apart holding your torso up at arm's length.

2 While inhaling, lower yourself until your chest almost touches the floor.

3 Exhale as you use your pectoral muscles to press your upper body back up to the starting position.

Variations: To make this exercise easier, you can bend your legs at the knees to take off resistance, or perform the exercise against the wall instead of the floor. To make this more difficult and increase resistance, you can place your feet at a high surface such as a bench. This also targets the upper chest.

Incline Bench Flies

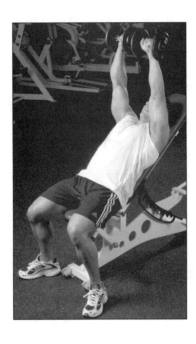 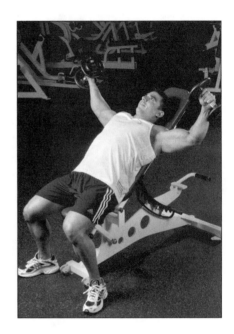

1 Lie back on an incline bench with a dumbbell on each hand on top of your thighs. The palms of your hand will be facing each other.

2 Using your thighs to help you get the dumbbells up, clean the dumbbells one arm at a time, and hold them at shoulder width. Rotate your wrists forward so the palms of your hands face away from you.

3 Bend your elbows slightly to prevent stress at the biceps tendon. Inhale while lowering your arms together in a wide arc until you feel a stretch on your chest. The arms should remain stationary as movement occurs at the shoulder joint.

4 Exhale and return your arms to the starting position using the same arc of motion. Hold this position for a second and repeat.

Variations: Varying the angle of the bench targets the upper chest at slightly different angles. Facing your palms together gives a slightly different stimulation.

Flat Bench Flies

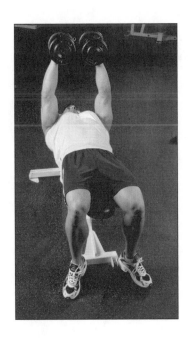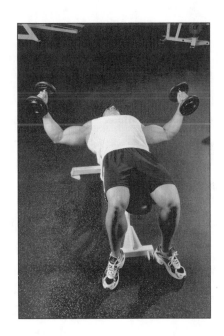

1 Lie down on a flat bench with a dumbbell on each hand on top of your thighs. The palms of your hands will be facing each other.

2 Repeat instructions for incline bench flies.

Standing Cable Crossovers

❶ For this exercise you will need access to a pulley machine. To get yourself into the starting position, place the pulleys above your head, select the proper resistance and hold the pulleys in each hand. Take a step forward of the imaginary straight line drawn between both pulleys while moving your arms straight out in front of you. Your torso will bend slightly forward from the waist.

❷ Bend your elbows slightly to prevent stress at the biceps tendon. Inhale and extend your arms straight out to the sides in a wide arc until you feel a stretch on your chest. Throughout the movement, the arms and torso should remain stationary; movement should occur only at the shoulder joint.

❸ Using the same arc of motion, exhale and return your arms to the starting position. Pause for a second at the apex of the movement and repeat.

Variations: You can vary the point where your arms meet.

Standing Cable Crossovers

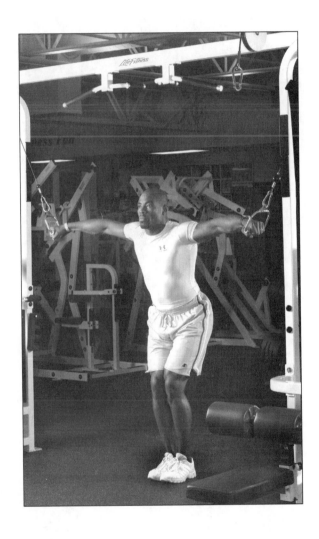

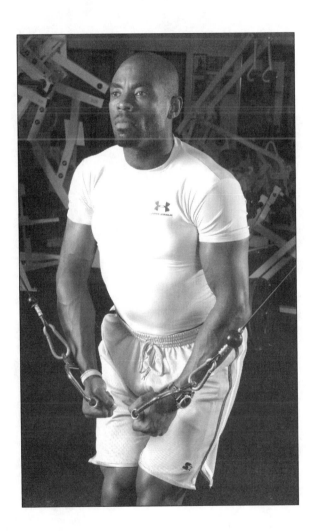

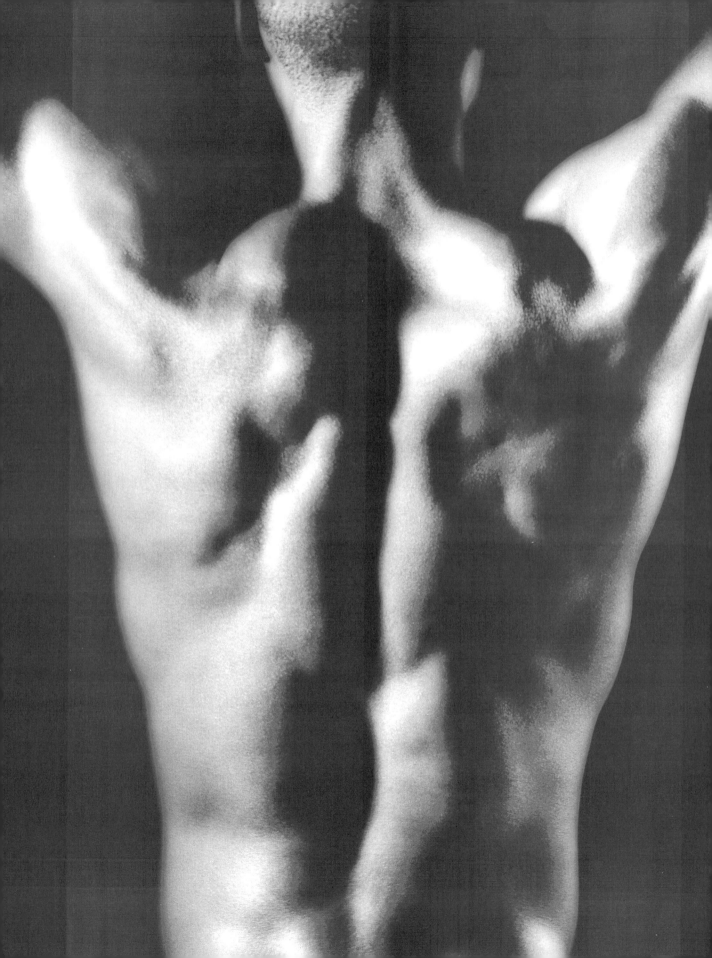

CHAPTER 8

Back Exercises

BASIC EXERCISES

Pull-down to Front
One Arm Dumbbell Rows
Pull-up to Front
Close Grip Chins
Neutral Grip Pull-ups

ISOLATION EXERCISES

Low Pulley Rows
Stiff-Arm Pull-downs

ALTERNATIVE EXERCISES

Close Grip Pull-downs (Basic)
Close Grip Pull-downs
*   with a V-Bar (Basic)*
Two Arm Rows (Basic)
Bent-Arm Pullovers for Back (Basic)
Bent Knee Deadlifts (Basic)

In this chapter we will cover the execution of all the back exercises presented in the routines of this program.

The back muscles are: the latissimus dorsi which provides back width; the middle back, which provides back thickness, and the lower back, which consists of the spinal erectors. In order to have a powerful-looking back, the size of the lats needs to be maximized to attain a wide look, and the middle back and lower back muscles must be thick. We will now cover the exercises used on this program and at the end of the chapter I will cover some additional useful exercises that can be used as well in lieu of the ones in the routines above.

Target Muscles Groups with Your Grip

There are three grips that we need to be concerned with. All three can be either pronated (with your palms up) or supernated (with your palms down). In addition, the close grip can be neutral.

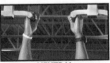 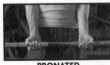 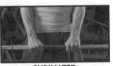

| NEUTRAL | PRONATED | SUPINATED |

Close Grip: This is where you grasp the bar with your hands 6 to 4 inches apart.

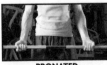 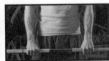 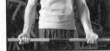 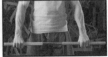

| PRONATED | SUPINATED | PRONATED | SUPINATED |

Medium Grip: For this grip, you grasp the bar with your hands just within or at shoulder width.

Wide Grip: This is where you grasp the bar with your hands 4 to 6 inches beyond shoulder width.

Pull-down to Front

GRIP: *Wide grip, medium grip, close grip*

1 Sit down on a pulldown machine with a wide bar attached to the top pulley. Adjust the knee pad of the machine to fit your height. These pads will prevent your body from being raised by the resistance attached to the bar.

2 Grab the bar with the palms facing forward using the prescribed grip. For a wide grip, your hands need to be spaced out at a distance wider than your shoulder width. For a medium grip, your hands need to be spaced out at a distance equal to your shoulder width, and for a close grip at a distance smaller than your shoulder width.

3 As you have both arms extended in front of you holding the bar at the chosen grip width, bring your torso back around 30 degrees or so while creating a curvature in your lower back and sticking your chest out. This is your starting position.

4 As you breathe out, bring the bar down until it touches your upper chest by drawing the shoulders and the upper arms down and back. Concentrate on squeezing the back muscles once you reach the full contracted position. The upper torso should remain stationary and only the arms should move.

The forearms should do no work other than holding the bar; therefore do not try to pull down the bar using the forearms.

5 After a second in the contracted position, while breathing in, slowly raise the bar back to the starting position when your arms are fully extended and the lats are fully stretched.

6 Repeat this motion for the prescribed number of repetitions.

Variations: The behind the neck variation is not recommended as it can be hard on the rotator cuff due to the hyperextension created by bringing the bar behind the neck.

Pull-down to Front

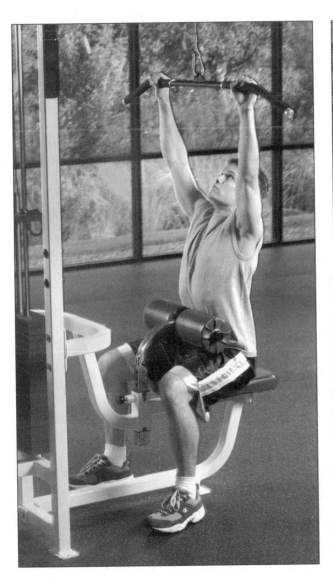
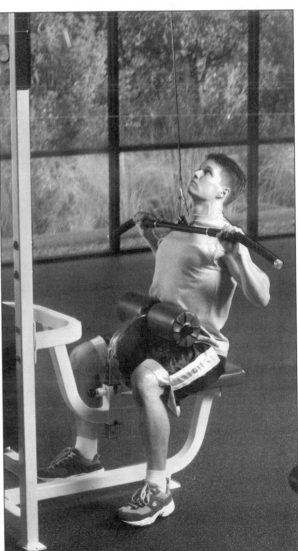

One Arm Dumbbell Rows

❶ Choose a flat bench and place a dumbbell on each side of it.

❷ Place the right knee on top of the end of the bench, bend your torso forward from the waist until your upper body is parallel to the floor, and place your right hand on the other end of the bench for support.

❸ Use the left hand to pick up the dumbbell on the floor and hold the weight while keeping your lower back straight. The palm of the hand should be facing your torso. This will be your starting position.

❹ Pull the resistance straight up to the side of your chest, keeping your upper arm close to your side and keeping the torso stationary. Breathe out as you perform this step. Also, make sure that the action is performed with the back muscles and not the arms.

❺ Lower the resistance straight down to the starting position. Breathe in as you perform this step.

❻ Repeat the movement for the specified amount of repetitions.

❼ Switch sides and repeat again with the other arm.

Variations: One-arm rows can also be performed using a high pulley or a low pulley instead of a dumbbell.

One Arm Dumbbell Rows

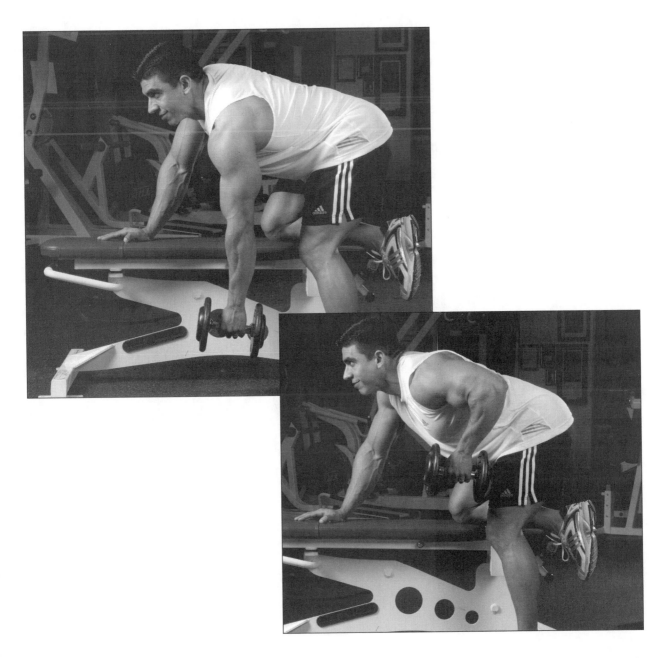

Pull-up to Front

GRIP: *Wide grip, medium grip, close grip*

1 Grab the pull-up bar with the palms facing forward using the prescribed grip. For a wide grip, your hands need to be spaced out at a distance wider than your shoulder width. For a medium grip, your hands need to be spaced out at a distance equal to your shoulder width, and for a close grip at a distance smaller than your shoulder width.

2 As you have both arms extended in front of you holding the bar at the chosen grip width, bring your torso back 30 degrees or so while creating a curvature in your lower back and sticking your chest out. This is your starting position.

3 As you breathe out, pull your torso up until the bar touches your upper chest by drawing the shoulders and the upper arms down and back. Concentrate on squeezing the back muscles once you reach the full contracted position. The upper torso should remain stationary as it moves through space and only the arms should move. The forearms should do no work other than holding the bar.

4 After a second on the contracted position, while breathing in, slowly lower your torso back to the starting position when your arms are fully extended and the lats are fully stretched.

5 Repeat this motion for the prescribed amount of repetitions.

Variations: If you are new at this exercise and do not have the strength to perform it, use a pull-up assist machine if available. These machines use weight to help you push your body weight. Otherwise, a spotter holding your legs can help. If none of these two options are available, then substitute a pull-down. On the other hand, more advanced lifters can add weight to the exercise by using a weight belt that allows the addition of weighted plates. Also, the behind-the-neck variation is not recommended as it can be hard on the rotator cuff due to the hyperextension created by bringing the bar behind the neck.

Pull-up to Front

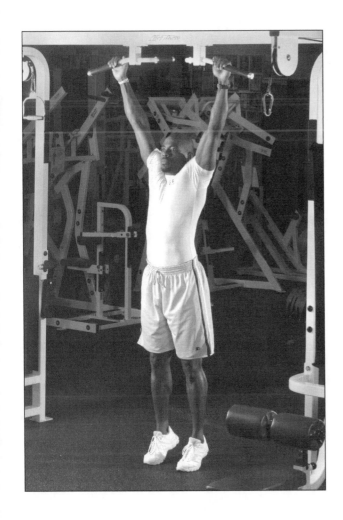 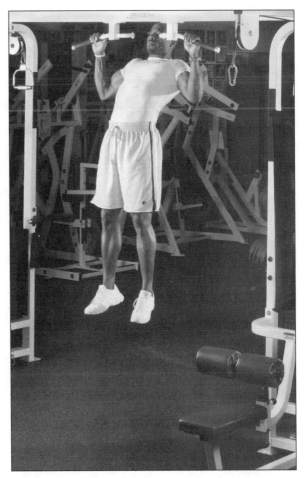

Close Grip Chins

GRIP: *Reverse grip*

1 Grab the pull-up bar with the palms facing your torso and a grip closer than the shoulder width.

2 As you have both arms extended in front of you holding the bar at the chosen grip width, bring your torso back 30 degrees or so while creating a curvature in your lower back and sticking your chest out. This is your starting position.

3 As you breathe out, pull your torso up until the bar touches your upper chest by drawing the shoulders and the upper arms down and back. Concentrate on squeezing the back muscles once you reach the full contracted position and keep the elbows close to your body. The upper torso should remain stationary; only the arms should move. The forearms should do no work other than holding the bar.

4 After a second in the contracted position, while breathing in, slowly lower your torso back to the starting position with your arms fully extended and the lats fully stretched.

5 Repeat this motion for the prescribed amount of repetitions.

Variations: If you are new at this exercise and do not have the strength to perform it, use a pull-up assist machine if available. These machines use weight to help you push your body weight. Otherwise, a spotter holding your legs can help. If none of these two options are available, then substitute a pull-down with a reverse grip. On the other hand, more advanced lifters can add weight to the exercise by using a weight belt that allows the addition of weighted plates.

Close Grip Chins

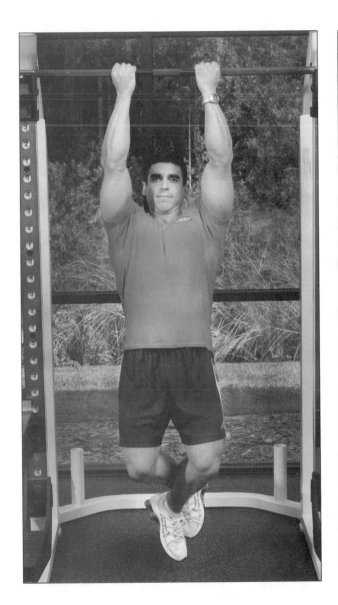
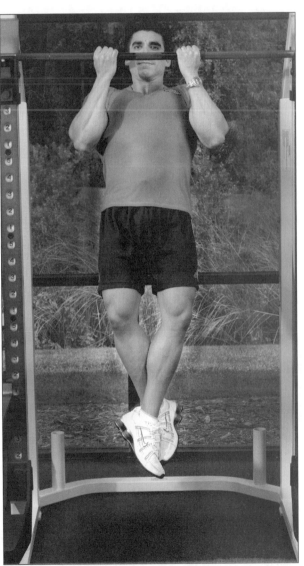

Neutral Grip Pull-ups

❶ For this exercise you will need access to a V-bar (the triangular bar with two handles used for the low pulley rows) and a pull-up bar. Start by placing the middle of the V-bar in the middle of the pull-up bar. The V-bar handles will be facing down so that you can hang from the pull-up bar through the use of the handles. Once you securely place the V-bar, take hold of the bar from each side and hang from it. Stick your chest out and lean yourself back slightly in order to better engage the lats. This will be your starting position.

❷ Using your lats, pull your torso up while leaning your head back slightly so that you do not hit yourself with the chin-up bar. Continue until your chest nearly touches the V-bar. Exhale as you execute this motion.

❸ After a second hold in the contracted position, slowly lower your body back to the starting position as you breathe in.

❹ Repeat for the prescribed number of repetitions.

Variations: If you are new at this exercise and do not have the strength to perform it, use a pull-up assist machine if available. These machines use weight to help you push your body weight. Otherwise, a spotter holding your legs can help. If none of these two options are available, then substitute a pull-down using a V-bar attachment. On the other hand, more advanced lifters can add weight to the exercise by using a weight belt that allows the addition of weighted plates.

Neutral Grip Pull-ups

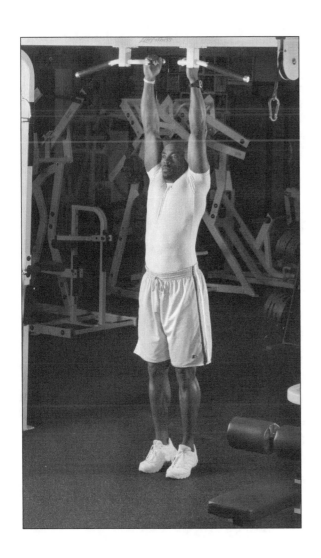
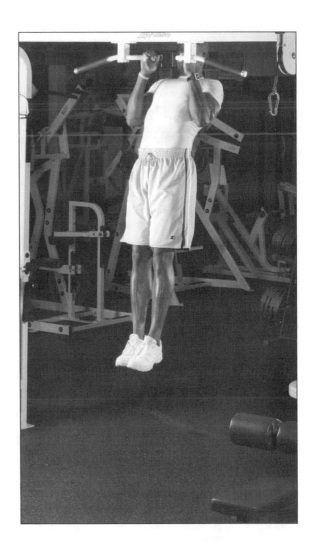

Bent Knee Deadlifts

1 Stand facing a loaded barbell.

2 While keeping the back as straight as possible, bend your knees, bend forward and grasp the bar using a medium (shoulder width) overhand grip (pronated grip: palms facing down). This will be the starting position of the exercise. (Note: You can use wrist wraps for this exercise.)

3 While holding the bar, start the lift by pushing with your legs while simultaneously getting your torso to the upright position as you breathe out. In the upright position, stick your chest out and contract the back by bringing the shoulder blades back. Think of how the soldiers look when they are standing at attention.

4 Go back slowly to the starting position by bending at the knees while simultaneously leaning the torso forward at the waist while keeping the back straight and breathing in. When the weights on the bar touch the floor you are back at the starting position and ready to perform another repetition.

5 Perform the number of repetitions prescribed in the program.

Caution: This is not an exercise to be taken lightly. If you have back issues, substitute a rowing motion instead. If you have a healthy back, ensure perfect form and never slouch the back forward as this can cause back injury. Be cautious as well with the weight used; in case of doubt, use less weight rather than more.

Variations: Dumbbells can be used as well though I find the bar version easier to perform as with dumbbells it is hard to find the correct groove of the exercise.

Notes: When adding weight, be very cautious and ensure that you can handle the load. While very effective, additional weight can make this exercise very dangerous to the lower back due to slight changes in form.

Bent Knee Deadlifts

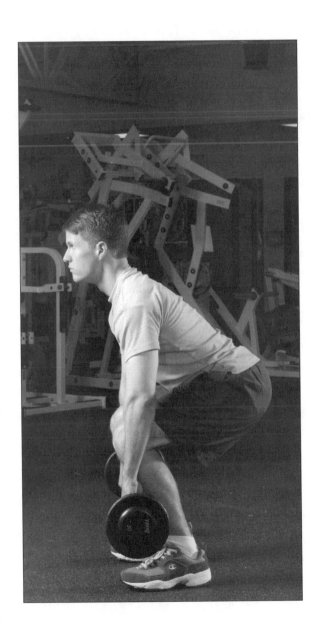 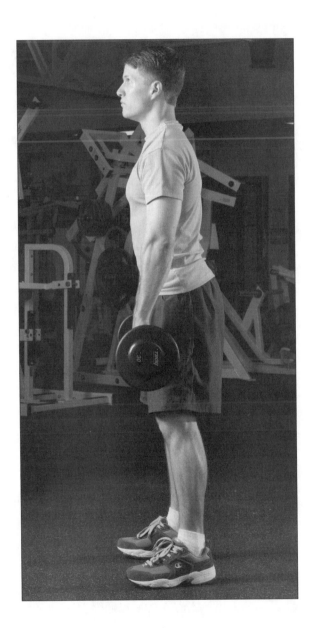

Low Pulley Rows

❶ For this exercise you will need access to a low pulley row machine with a V-bar (bar that enables you to have a neutral grip where the palms of your hands face each other). To get into the starting position, first sit down on the machine and place your feet on the front platform or crossbar provided, making sure that your knees are slightly bent and not locked.

❷ Lean over without arching your back forward and grab the handles. With your arms extended pull back until your torso is at a 90-degree angle with your legs. Your back should be slightly arched and your chest should be sticking out. You should be feeling a nice stretch on your lats as you hold the bar in front of you. This is the starting position of the exercise.

❸ Keeping the torso stationary, pull the handles back towards your torso while keeping the arms close to it until you touch the abdominals. Breathe out as you perform that movement. At that point you should be squeezing your back muscles hard. Hold that contraction for a second and slowly go back to the original position while breathing in.

❹ Repeat for the recommended amount of repetitions.

Caution: Avoid swinging your torso back and forth as you can cause lower back injury by doing so.

Variations: You can use a straight bar instead of a V-bar and perform with a pronated grip (palms facing down-forward) or a supinated grip (palms facing up—reverse grip).

Low Pulley Rows

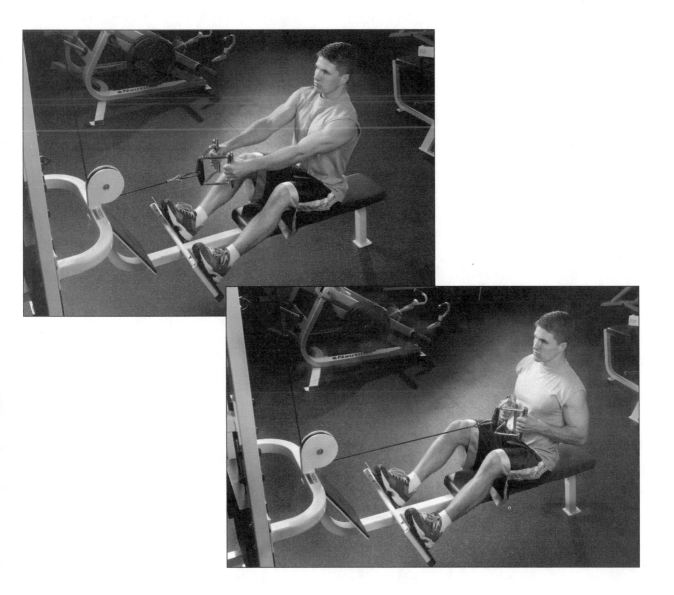

Stiff-Arm Pull-downs

1 For this exercise you will need access to a high pulley and a rope attached to it. You will start by grabbing the rope from the top pulley and stepping backward two feet or so.

2 Bend your torso forward at the waist by about 30 degrees with your arms fully extended, with a slight bend at the elbows. If your arms are not fully extended then you need to step back a bit more until they are. Once your arms are fully extended and your torso is slightly bent at the waist, tighten the lats and then you are ready to begin.

3 While keeping the arms straight, pull the rope down by contracting the lats until your hands are next to the sides of the thighs. Breathe out as you perform this step.

4 While keeping the arms straight, go back to the starting position while breathing in.

5 Repeat for the recommended amount of repetitions.

Variations: You can also use a straight bar for variety, in which case you need to grab it using a pronated grip (palms down).

Stiff-Arm Pull-downs

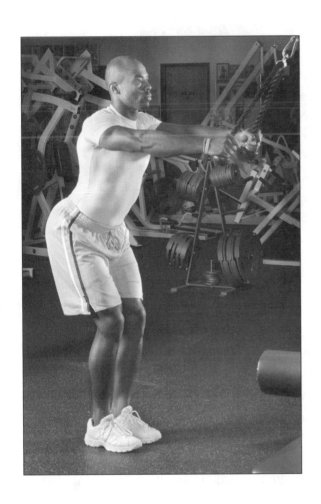 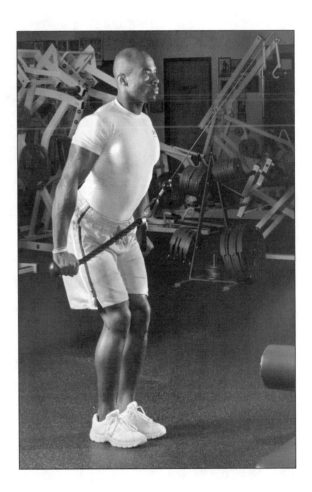

Close Grip Pull-downs

GRIP: *Palms facing your body*

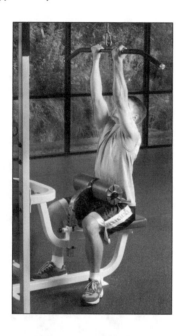
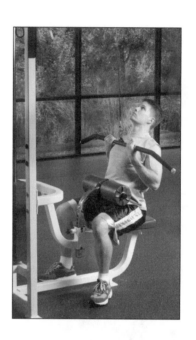

❶ Sit down on a pull-down machine with a wide bar attached to the top pulley. Adjust the knee pad of the machine. Grasp the pull-down bar with palms facing your torso and a grip narrower than shoulder width.

❷ Extended both arms in front of you holding the bar and pull your torso back, creating a curvature in your lower back and a proud chest. This is your starting position.

❸ Exhale and pull the bar down, touching your upper chest and drawing the shoulders and the upper arms down and back. Squeeze your back muscles once you reach the fully contracted position, and make sure to keep your elbows close to your body. Only your arms should move, and the forearms should only be holding the bar.

❹ Hold a second in the contracted position, then inhale while slowly bringing the bar back to the starting position where your arms are fully extended and the lats are fully stretched.

Close Grip Pull-downs with a V-bar

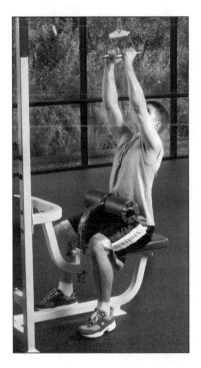 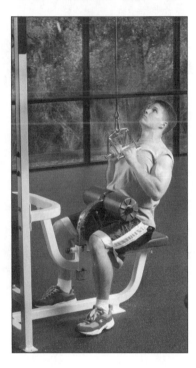

❶ Sit down at a pulldown machine with a V-bar attached to the top pulley. Adjust the knee pad of the machine. Grab the V-bar with the palms facing each other and stick your chest out and lean back slightly to better engage the lats.

❷ Exhale while pulling the bar down, keeping your torso stationary. Continue pulling until your chest nearly touches the V-bar.

❸ Hold at the contracted position, then inhale, slowly bringing the bar back to the starting position.

Two Arm Rows

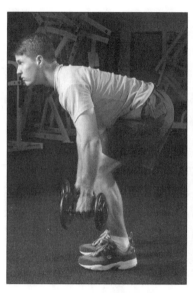 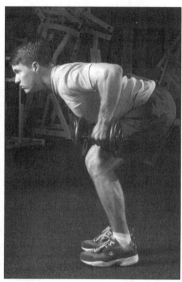

1 Hold a dumbbell in each hand, with your palms facing your torso. Bend your knees slightly and push your torso forward by bending at the waist, keeping the back straight until it is almost parallel to the floor. Your head should be up, and the weights should hang with your arms perpendicular to the floor.

2 While holding the torso stationary, lift the dumbbells to your sides as you exhale, keeping your elbows close to your body and not using your forearms for anything but positioning. At the top of the contraction, squeeze your back muscles and hold for a second.

3 Slowly lower the weights again to the starting position.

Caution: This exercise is not recommended for people with back problems. Instead, use a low pulley row. Maintain perfect form for this exercise and never slouch the back forward as this can cause back injury. If you are unfamiliar with this exercise, use less weight rather than more.

Variations: You can perform the same exercise using a low pulley instead with a V-bar.

Bent-Arm Pullovers for Back

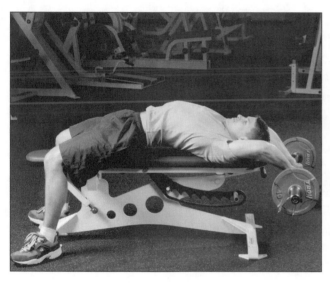

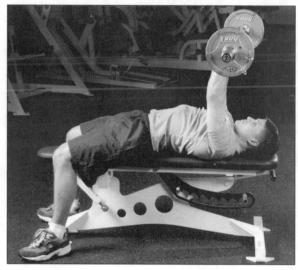

❶ Lie on a flat bench with either an E-Z bar or a straight bar placed on the floor behind your head and your feet flat on the floor.

❷ Using a medium overhand (pronated) grip, grasp the bar behind you and raise, keeping your arms bent.

❸ Bring the bar over the head to the chest as you exhale.

❹ Now start bringing the bar back down slowly to the starting position (without letting the weights touch the floor) as you inhale.

❺ Once you feel a stretch on your lats, start bringing the weight back up and repeat for the recommended number of repetitions.

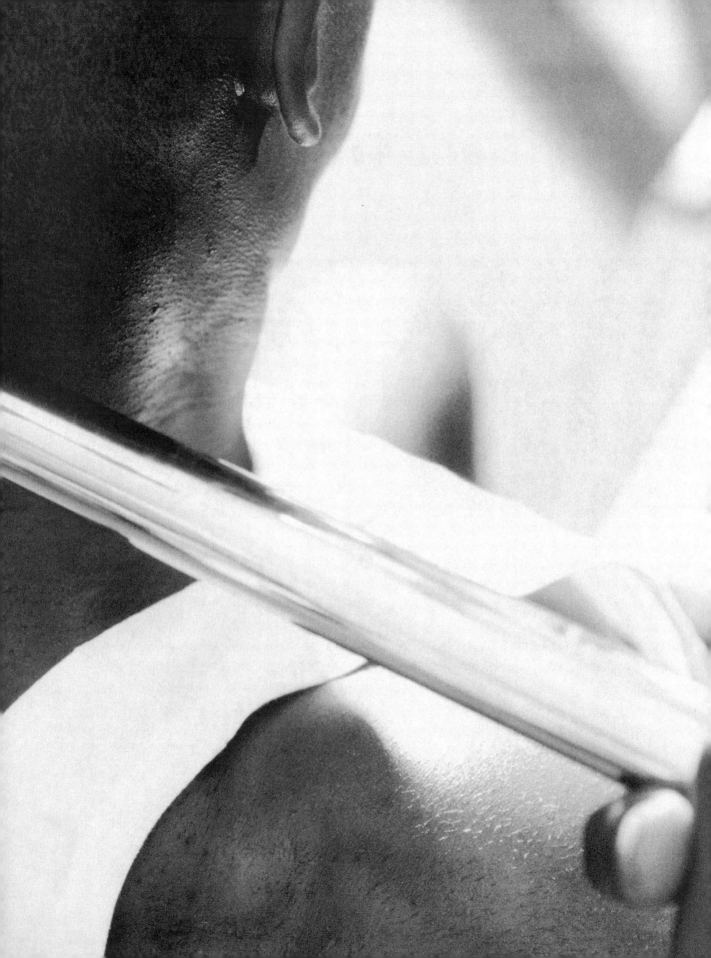

CHAPTER 9

Shoulder Exercises

BASIC EXERCISES

Dumbbell Shoulder Press

Seated Military Press

Upright Rows

ISOLATION EXERCISES

Bent-over Lateral Raises

Bent Arm Bent-over Rows

Incline One Arm Laterals

Lateral Raises

ALTERNATIVE EXERCISES

Front Raises (Isolation)

Bent-over Laterals on
    Incline Bench (Isolation)

Rear Delt Rows (Isolation)

In this chapter we will cover the execution of all the shoulder exercises presented in the routines of this program.

The shoulders are a muscle group that consists of three main parts; the anterior (front) deltoid, the lateral (side) deltoid and the posterior (rear) deltoids. In order to have powerful looking shoulders and a wide, thick look, the size of the three heads needs to be maximized. We will now cover the exercises used on this program and at the end of the chapter I will cover some additional useful exercises that can be used as well in lieu of the ones in the routines above.

Dumbbell Shoulder Press

1 Grab a couple of dumbbells and sit on a military press bench or a utility bench that has a back support on it as you place the dumbbells upright on top of your thighs.

2 Clean the dumbbells up one at a time by using your thighs to bring the dumbbells up to shoulder height at each side.

3 Rotate the wrists so that the palms of your hands are facing forward. This is your starting position.

4 As you exhale, push the dumbbells up until they touch at the top.

5 After a second pause, slowly come down back to the starting position as you inhale.

6 Repeat for the recommended number of repetitions.

Variations: You can perform the exercise standing or sitting on a regular flat bench. For people with lower back problems, the version described is the recommended one. You can also perform the exercise as Arnold Schwarzenegger used to do it, which is to start holding the dumbbells with a supinated grip (palms facing you) in front of your shoulders and then, as you start pushing up, you align the dumbbells in the starting position described in step 3 by rotating your wrists and touching the dumbbells at the top as you come down, then go back to the starting position by rotating the wrist throughout the lowering portion until the palms of your hands are facing you. This variation is called the Arnold Press. However, it is not recommended if you have rotator cuff problems.

Dumbbell Shoulder Press

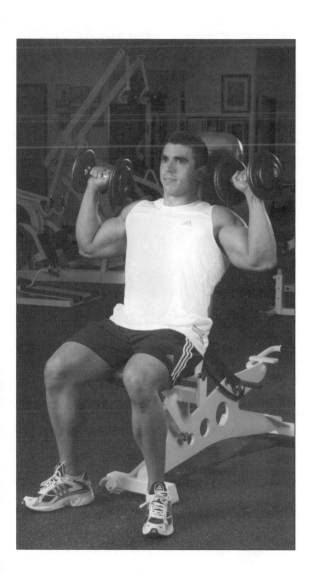 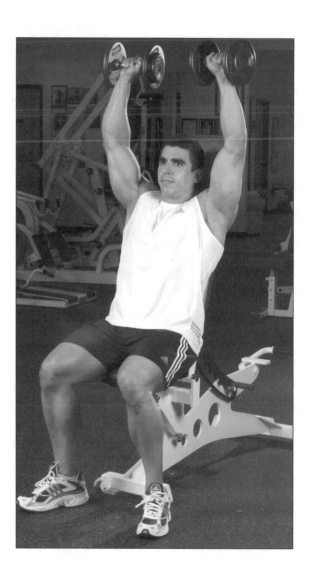

Seated Military Press

❶ Sit on a military press bench with a bar behind your head and either have a spotter give you the bar (better on the rotator cuff this way) or pick it up yourself carefully with a pronated grip (palms facing forward). Your grip should be wider than shoulder width and it should create a 90-degree angle between the forearm and the upper arm as the barbell goes down.

❷ Once you pick up the barbell with the correct grip length, lift the bar up over your head by locking your arms. Hold at about shoulder level and slightly in front of your head. This is your starting position.

❸ Lower the bar down to the collarbone slowly as you inhale.

❹ Lift the bar back up to the starting position as you exhale.

❺ Repeat for the recommended amount of repetitions.

Variations: This exercise can also be performed standing but those with lower back problems are better off performing this seated variety. The behind-the-neck variation is not recommended as it can be hard on the rotator cuff due to the hyperextension created by bringing the bar behind the neck. Behind-the-neck presses can cause injury.

Seated Military Press

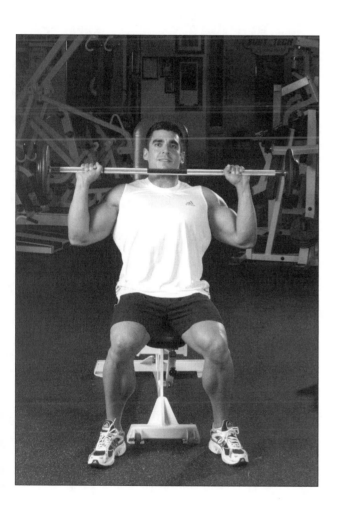
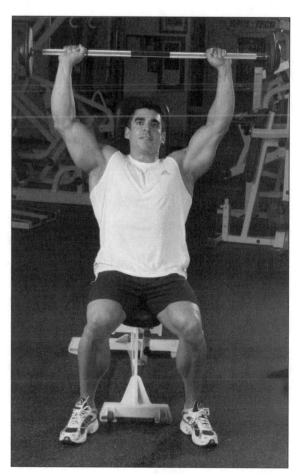

Upright Rows

1 Grasp an E-Z curl bar (my preference) or a barbell with a pronated (palms forward) grip that is slightly less than shoulder width. The bar should be resting on top of your thighs. Your arms should be extended with a slight bend at the elbows and your back should be straight. This will be your starting position.

2 As you breathe out, use your side shoulders to lift the bar as you exhale. The bar should be close to the body as you move it up. Continue to lift it until it nearly touches your chin. Keep your torso stationary and pause for a second at the top of the movement.

3 Lower the bar back down slowly to the starting position. Inhale as you perform this portion of the movement.

4 Repeat for the recommended amount of repetitions.

Caution: Be very careful how much weight you use in this exercise. Too much weight leads to bad form, which in turn can cause shoulder injury. I've seen this too many times, so please, no jerking, swinging, and cheating. Also, if you suffer from shoulder problems, you may want to stay away from upright rows and substitute by some form of lateral raises.

Variations: This exercise can also be performed using a straight bar attached to a low pulley and it can also be performed using dumbbells, though this exercise should be reserved for the most advanced people that are familiar with correct execution.

Notes: Be extremely careful to use perfect form, because sloppy form often leads to rotator cuff injuries.

Upright Rows

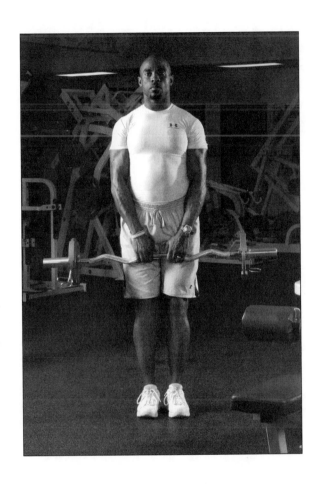 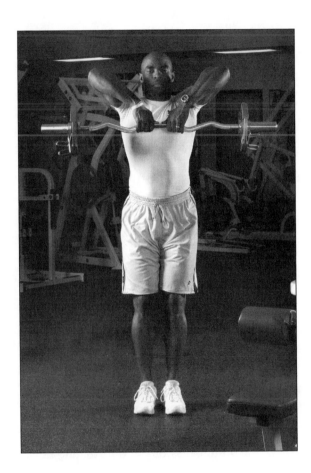

Bent-over Lateral Raises

1 Place a couple of dumbbells parallel to and in front of a flat bench.

2 Sit on the end of the bench with your legs together and the dumbbells behind your calves.

3 Bend at the waist while keeping the back straight in order to pick up the dumbbells. The palms of your hands should be facing each other as you pick them. This will be your starting position.

4 Keeping your torso forward and stationary, and the arms slightly bent at the elbows, lift the dumbbells straight to the side until both arms are parallel to the floor. Exhale as you lift the weights. (Note: avoid swinging the torso or bringing the arms back rather than to the side.)

5 After a 1-second contraction at the top, slowly lower the dumbbells back to the starting position.

6 Repeat the recommended number of repetitions.

Variations: This exercise can also be performed standing but those with lower back problems are better off performing this seated version.

Bent-over Lateral Raises

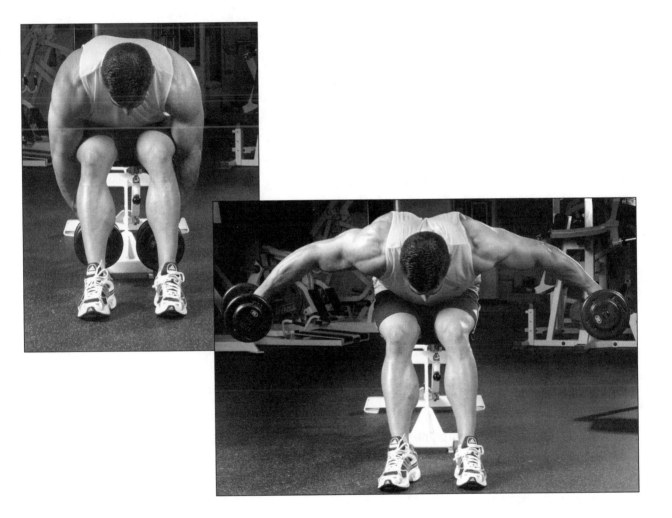

Bent Arm Bent-over Rows

1 Place a couple of dumbbells parallel to and in front of a flat bench.

2 Sit on the end of the bench with your legs together and the dumbbells behind your calves.

3 Bend at the waist while keeping the back straight in order to pick up the dumbbells. The palms of your hands should be facing each other as you pick them up.

4 Bend at the elbows until there is a 90-degree angle formed between the forearm and the upper arm. This will be your starting position.

5 Keeping your torso forward and stationary, and the arms bent at a 90-degree angle at the elbows, lift the dumbbells straight to the side until both upper arms are parallel to the floor. (Note: The forearms should be pointing straight to the floor in the contracted position.) Exhale as you lift the weights. (Note: avoid swinging the torso or bringing the arms back as rather than to the side.)

6 After a 1-second contraction at the top, slowly lower the dumbbells back to the starting position.

7 Repeat the recommended amount of repetitions.

Variations: This exercise can also be performed standing, but those with lower back problems are better off performing this seated variety.

Bent-Arm Bent-over Rows

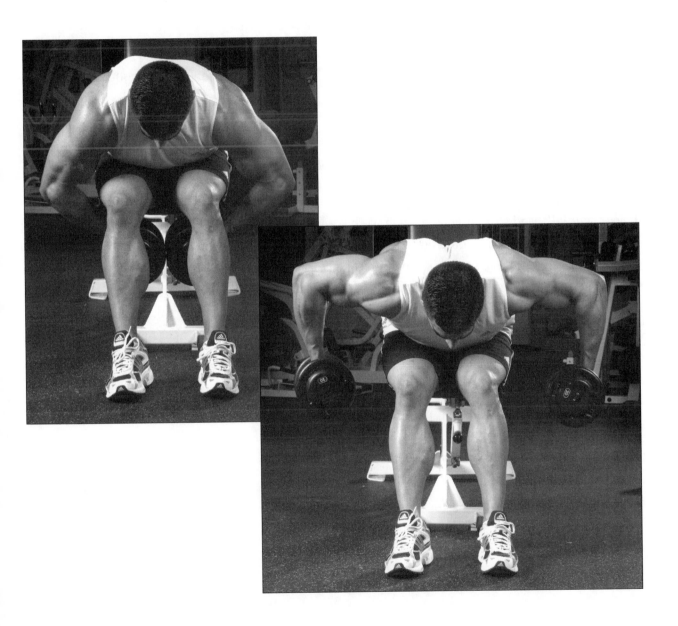

Incline One Arm Laterals

1 For this exercise you will need one dumbbell and a sturdy object to hold onto such as one of the beams on a squat rack or a stationary handle provided by some pulley machines. Start by grabbing the dumbbell with your right arm and using the left arm to hold on to the sturdy object.

2 Place your feet close to the imaginary line below your left hand so that you can lean to the side towards the opposite direction. The right hand should be pointing straight down to the floor while holding the dumbbell. This will be your starting position.

3 While keeping the torso stationary (no swinging) and leaning to the side, lift the dumbbell to your side with a slight bend in the elbow and the hands slightly tilted forward as if pouring water in a glass. Continue to raise your arm until it is parallel to the floor. Exhale as you execute this movement and pause for a second at the top.

4 Lower the dumbbell slowly to the starting position as you inhale.

5 Repeat for the recommended number of repetitions. When done with the right arm, perform with the left.

Variations: This exercise can also be performed using cables.

Incline One Arm Laterals

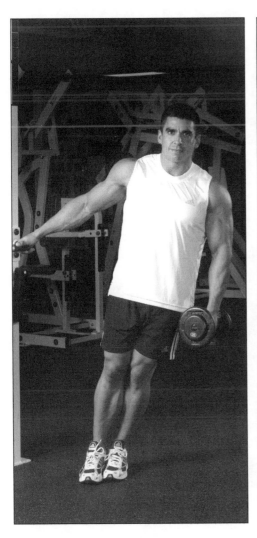
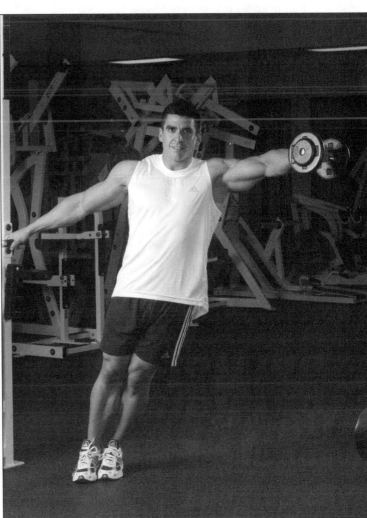

Lateral Raises

❶ Pick up a couple of dumbbells and stand with a straight torso and the dumbbells by your side at arm's length with the palms of the hand facing you. This will be your starting position.

❷ While keeping the torso stationary (no swinging), lift the dumbbells to your sides with a slight bend in the elbow and the hands slightly tilted forward as if pouring water in a glass. Continue to raise until your arms until they are parallel to the floor. Exhale as you execute this movement and pause for a second at the top.

❸ Lower the dumbbells slowly to the starting position as you inhale.

❹ Repeat for the recommended number of repetitions.

Variations: This exercise can also be performed sitting down.

Lateral Raises

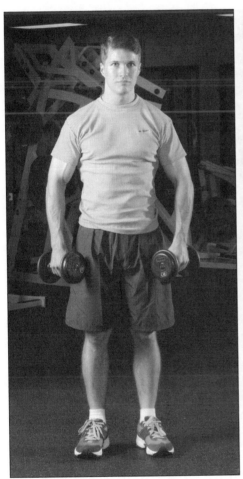 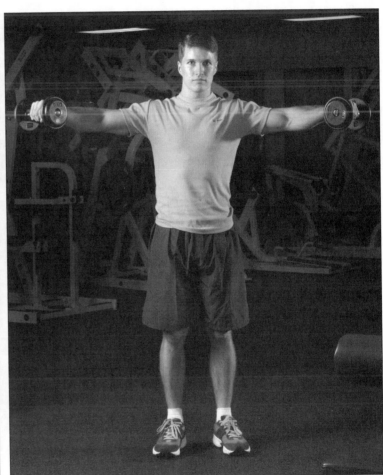

Front Raises

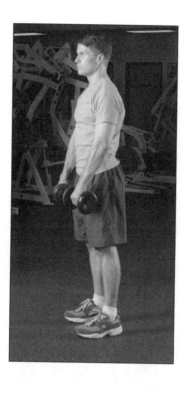 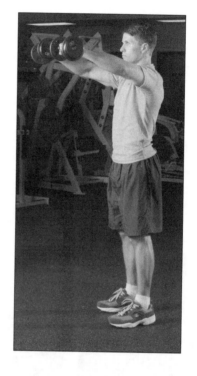

❶ Stand with a straight torso and the dumbbells resting in front of your thighs with the palms of your hand facing you.

❷ While standing still, lift the dumbbells straight to the front, with a slight bend on the elbow and the palms of the hands facing down. While exhaling, continue until your arms are parallel to the floor. Pause for a second at the top.

❸ As you inhale, lower the dumbbells slowly to the starting position.

Variations: This exercise can also be performed by one hand alone, as well as alternating. You could also use a barbell.

Bent-over Laterals on Incline Bench

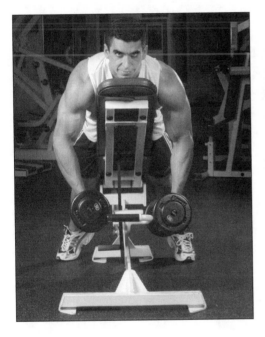 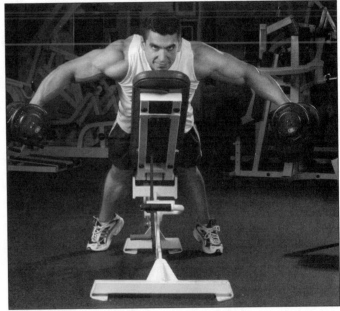

❶ Place a couple of dumbbells to the sides of an incline bench. Sit on the bench facing the incline pad with your legs to your sides behind the dumbbells. Pick up the dumbbells. The palms of your hands should be facing each other.

❷ Keeping your torso still on the incline pad and your arms slightly bent at the elbows, exhale as you lift the dumbbells straight to the side until both arms are parallel to the floor.

❸ After a one-second contraction at the top, slowly lower the dumbbells back to the starting position.

Rear Delt Rows

1 Choose a flat bench and place a dumbbell on each side of it. Place your right knee on top of the end of the bench, and bend your torso forward from the waist until your upper body is parallel to the floor. Place your right hand on the other end of the bench for support.

2 Use your left hand to pick up the dumbbell and hold the weight. Keep your lower back straight. The palm of the hand should be facing behind you and your arm should be extended.

3 While standing still, exhale and pull the dumbbell straight up by the side of your chest, keeping your upper arm away from your torso. As you go up, the elbow will bend out. Make sure that the action is performed with your back muscles and not your arms.

4 After a second pause at the top contraction, inhale, and lower the dumbbell to the starting position.

5 Repeat the movement for the specified number of repetitions.

6 Switch sides and repeat again with the other arm.

Variations: One-arm rear delt rows can also be performed using a high pulley or a low pulley instead of a dumbbell.

Rear Delt Rows

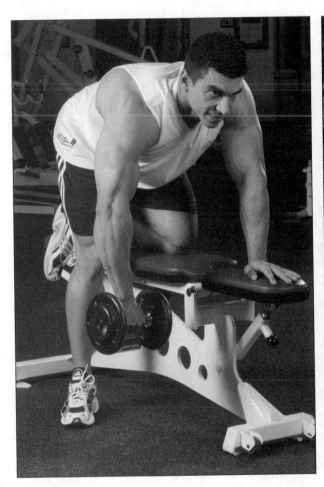
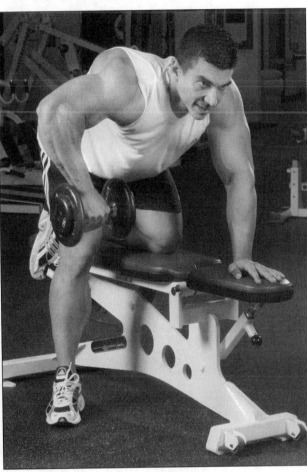

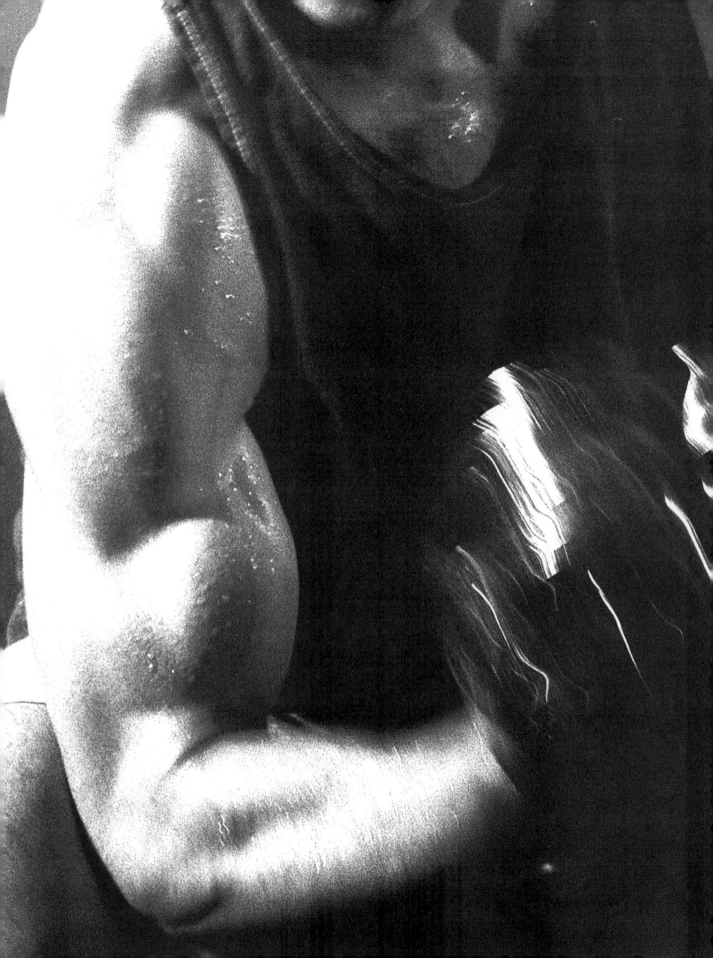

CHAPTER 10

Biceps Exercises

BASIC EXERCISES

Neutral Grip Chin-Ups

Close Grip Chin-Ups

ISOLATION EXERCISES

Incline Dumbbell Curls

Concentration Curls

Dumbbell Hammer Curls

Dumbbell Preacher Curls

E-Z Curls

E-Z Preacher Curls

E-Z Reverse Curls

ALTERNATIVE EXERCISES

High Pulley One Arm
    Cable Curls (Basic)

Dumbbell Curls (Isolation)

E-Z Reverse
    Preacher Curls (Isolation)

In this chapter we will cover the execution of all the biceps exercises presented in the routines of this program.

The biceps are a very popular muscle group that consists of two heads originating at the shoulder and inserting below the elbow. When most people ask you to show a muscle, this is the one they are looking for. In order to have a powerful looking biceps, the height of the muscle needs to be maximized as well as the width. We will now cover the exercises used on this program and at the end of the chapter I will cover some additional useful exercises that can be used as well in lieu of the ones in the routines above.

Neutral Grip Chin-Ups

GRIP: *Palms facing each other*

❶ This is the same exercise as the neutral grip pull-ups described in the back section, except that this time we will be using it to target the biceps mainly. For this exercise you will need access to a V-bar (the triangular bar with two handles used for the low pulley rows) and a pull-up bar. Start by placing the middle of the V-bar in the middle of the pull-up bar. The V-Bar handles will be facing down so that you can hang from the pull-up bar through the use of the handles. Once you securely place the V-bar, take hold of the bar from each side and hang from it. Stick your chest out while keeping the torso as straight as possible in order to limit engagement of the lats and maximize biceps stimulation. This will be your starting position.

❷ Using your biceps, pull your torso up while leaning your head back slightly so that you do not hit yourself with the chin-up bar. Continue until your head nearly touches the V-bar and your biceps are contracted (there should be an angle less than 90-degrees between the upper arm and the lower arm). Exhale as you execute this motion.

❸ After a second hold in the contracted position, slowly lower your body back to the starting position as you breathe in.

❹ Repeat for the prescribed number of repetitions.

Variations: If you are new at this exercise and do not have the strength to perform it, use a pull-up assist machine if available. These machines use weight to help you push your body weight. Otherwise, a spotter holding your legs can help. If none of these two options are available, then substitute a pull-down using a v-bar attachment. On the other hand, more advanced lifters can add weight to the exercise by using a weight belt that allows the addition of weighted plates.

Neutral Grip Chin-Ups

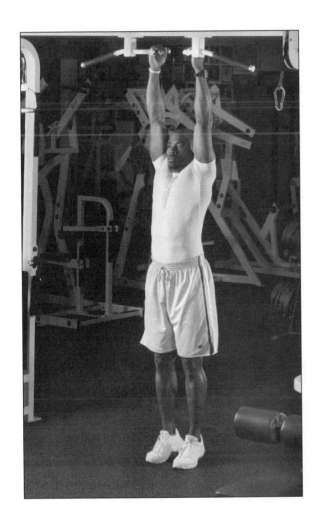
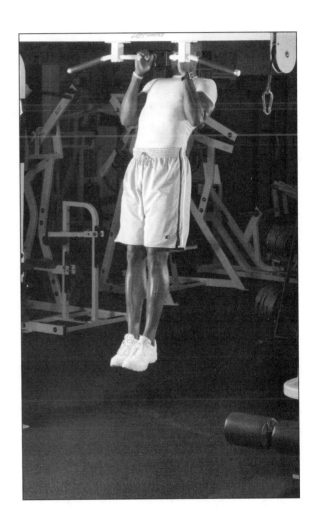

Close Grip Chin-Ups

GRIP: *Reverse grip*

① Same exercise as the one for back described earlier but emphasizing the biceps involvement. To perform it, grab the pull-up bar with the palms facing your torso and a grip closer than shoulder width.

② As you have both arms extended in front of you holding the bar at the chosen grip width, keep your torso as straight as possible while creating a curvature in your lower back and sticking your chest out. This is your starting position.

③ As you breathe out, pull your torso up until your head is at the level of the pull-up bar. Concentrate on using the biceps muscles to perform the movement. Keep the elbows close to your body. The upper torso should remain stationary as only the arms should move. The forearms should do no work other than hold the bar.

④ After a second in the contracted position, while breathing in, slowly lower your torso back to the starting position with your arms are fully extended and the lats are fully stretched.

⑤ Repeat this motion for the prescribed number of repetitions.

Variations: If you are new at this exercise and do not have the strength to perform it, use a pull-up assist machine if available. These machines use weight to help you push your body weight. Otherwise, a spotter holding your legs can help. If none of these two options are available, then substitute the a pull-down with a reverse grip. On the other hand, more advanced lifters can add weight to the exercise by using a weight belt that allows the addition of weighted plates.

Close Grip Chin-Ups

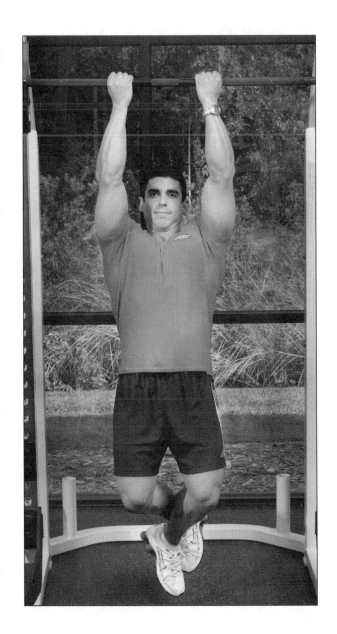
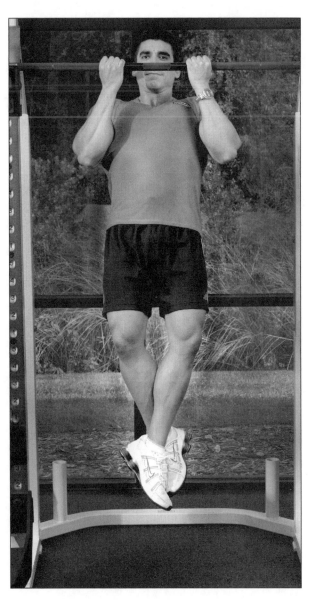

Incline Dumbbell Curls

❶ Sit down on an incline bench with a dumbbell in each hand held at arm's length. The elbows should be close to the torso.

❷ Rotate the palms of the hands until they are facing forward. This will be your starting position.

❸ While holding the upper arm stationary, curl the weights forward while contracting the biceps as you breathe out. Only the forearms should move. Continue the movement until your biceps are fully contracted and the dumbbells are at shoulder level. Hold the contracted position for a second.

❹ Slowly begin to bring the dumbbells back to starting position as your breathe in.

❺ Repeat for the recommended number of repetitions.

Incline Dumbbell Curls

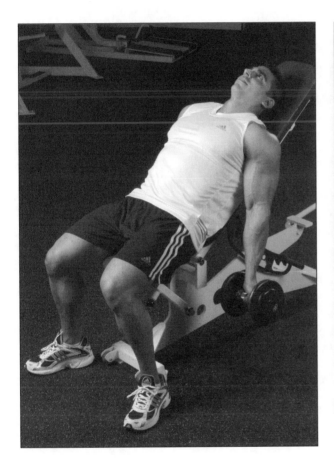
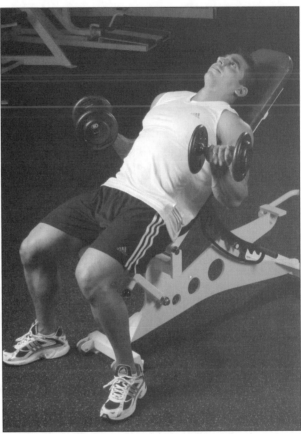

Concentration Curls

❶ Sit down on a flat bench with one dumbbell in front of you. Use the right arm to pick it up and place the back of that upper arm on top of your inner right thigh (about 3 1/2 inches away from the front of the knee). Rotate the palm of the hand until it is facing forward away from your thigh. Your arm should be fully extended and the dumbbell should be above the floor. This will be your starting position.

❷ While holding the upper arm stationary, curl the weight forward while contracting the biceps as you breathe out. Only the forearms should move. Continue the movement until your biceps are fully contracted and the dumbbell is at shoulder level. At the top of the movement make sure that the little finger of your arm is higher than your thumb. This guarantees a good contraction. Hold the contracted position for a second.

❸ Slowly begin to bring the dumbbells back to starting position as your breathe in. Avoid swinging motions at all times.

❹ Repeat for the recommended number of repetitions. Then repeat the movement with the left arm.

Variations: This exercise can be performed standing with the torso bent forward and the arm in front of you. In this case, no leg support is used for the back of your arm so you will need to make extra effort to ensure no movement of the upper arm. This is a more challenging version of the exercise and is not recommended for people with lower back problems.

Concentration Curls

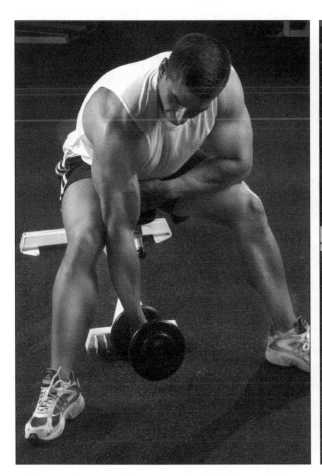

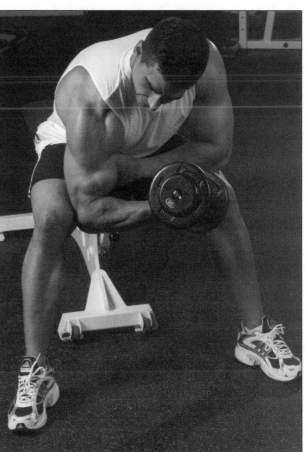

Dumbbell Hammer Curls

① Stand up with your torso upright and a dumbbell in each hand and arms fully extended. The elbows should be close to the torso.

② The palms of the hands should be facing your torso. This will be your starting position.

③ While holding the upper arm stationary, curl the weights forward while contracting the biceps as you breathe out. Only the forearms should move. Continue the movement until your biceps are fully contracted and the dumbbells are at shoulder level. Hold the contracted position for a second.

④ Slowly begin to bring the dumbbells back to starting position as your breathe in.

⑤ Repeat for the recommended number of repetitions.

Variations: There are many possible variations for this movement. For instance, you can perform the exercise sitting down on a bench with or without back support and you can also perform it by alternating arms; first lift the right arm for one repetition, then the left, then the right, etc.

Dumbbell Hammer Curls

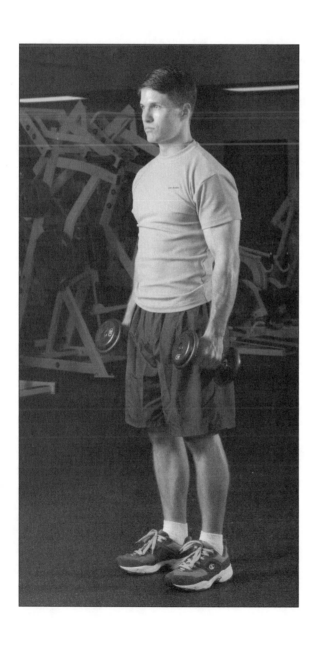 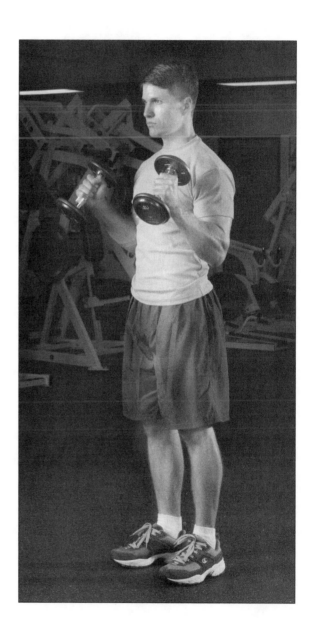

Dumbbell Preacher Curls

❶ To perform this movement you will either need a preacher bench or the top of an incline bench.

❷ Grab a dumbbell with the right arm and place the upper arm on top of the preacher bench or the incline bench. The dumbbell should be held at arms length. This will be your starting position.

❸ As you breathe in, slowly lower the dumbbell until your upper arm is extended and the biceps is fully stretched.

❹ As you exhale, use the biceps to curl the weight up until your biceps is fully contracted and the dumbbell is at shoulder height. Again, remember that to ensure full contraction you need to bring that last finger higher than the thumb.

❺ Repeat for the recommended number of repetitions. Then switch arms and repeat the movement.

Variations: You can perform this exercise also using a low pulley instead of a dumbbell. In this case you will need to position the bench in front of the pulley.

Dumbbell Preacher Curls

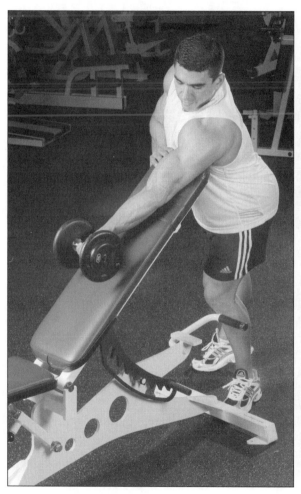
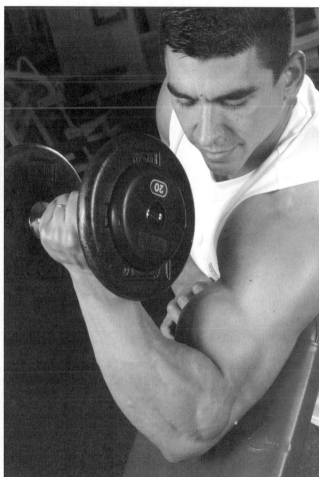

E-Z Curls

❶ Stand up with your torso upright while holding an E-Z curl bar at the wide outer handle. The palm of your hands should be facing forward and they should be slightly tilted inwards due to the shape of the bar. The elbows should be close to the torso. This will be your starting position.

❷ While holding the upper arms stationary, curl the weights forward while contracting the biceps as you breathe out. Only the forearms should move. Continue the movement until your biceps are fully contracted and the bar is at shoulder level. Hold the contracted position for a second.

❸ Slowly begin to bring the bar back to starting position as your breathe in.

❹ Repeat for the recommended amount of repetitions.

Variations: You can also perform this movement using an E-Z attachment hooked to a low pulley. This variation seems to really provide a good contraction at the top of the movement. You may also use the closer grip for variation purposes. Also, you can use a straight bar instead of the E-Z variation but straight bars place more stress on the wrist joint.

E-Z Curls

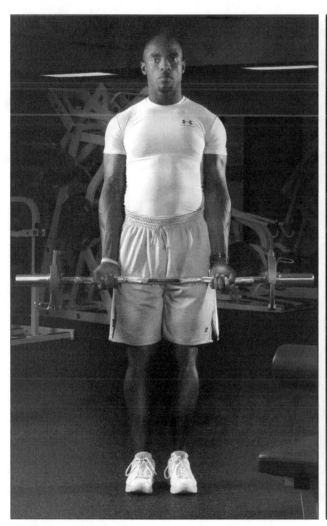 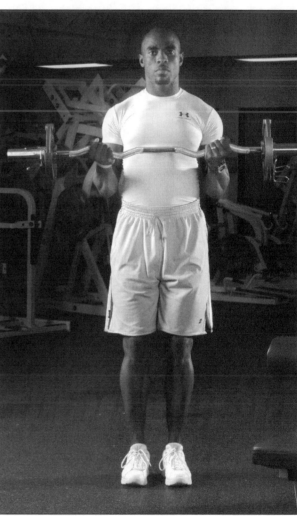

E-Z Preacher Curls

1 To perform this movement you will need a preacher bench and an E-Z bar. Grab the E-Z curl bar at the wide outer handle (either have someone hand you the bar, which is preferable, or grab the bar from the front bar rest provided by most preacher benches). The palms of your hands should be facing forward and they should be slightly tilted inwards due to the shape of the bar.

2 With the upper arms positioned against the preacher bench pad and the chest against it, hold the E-Z curl bar at shoulder height. This will be your starting position.

3 As you breathe in, slowly lower the bar until your upper arm is extended and the biceps is fully stretched.

4 As you exhale, use the biceps to curl the weight up until your biceps is fully contracted and the bar is at shoulder height.

5 Repeat for the recommended number of repetitions.

Variations: You can also perform this exercise using a low pulley with an E-Z bar attachment instead of an E-Z bar. In this case you will need to position the bench in front of the pulley. You may also use the closer grip for variation purposes. Also, you can use a straight bar instead of the E-Z variation but straight bars place more stress on the wrist joint.

E-Z Preacher Curls

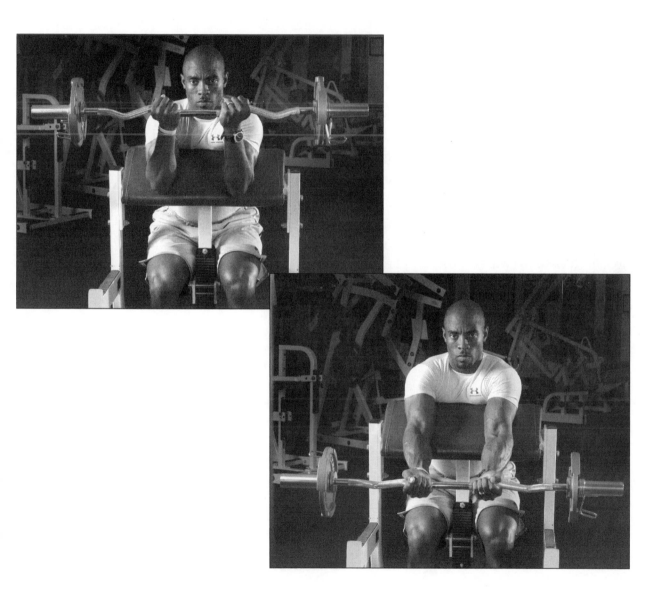

E-Z Reverse Curls

❶ Stand up with your torso upright while holding an E-Z curl bar at the wide outer handle. The palms of your hands should be facing down and they should be slightly tilted downwards to the shape of the bar (the thumb should be higher than the little finger). The elbows should be close to the torso. This will be your starting position.

❷ While holding the upper arms stationary, curl the weights toward you while contracting the biceps as you breathe out. Only the forearms should move. Continue the movement until your biceps are fully contracted and the bar is at shoulder level. Hold the contracted position for a second.

❸ Slowly begin to bring the bar back to starting position as your breathe in.

❹ Repeat for the recommended number of repetitions.

Variations: You can also perform this movement using an E-Z attachment hooked to a low pulley. This variation seems to really provide a good contraction at the top of the movement. Also, you can use a straight bar instead of the E-Z variation, but straight bars place more stress on the wrist joint.

E-Z Reverse Curls

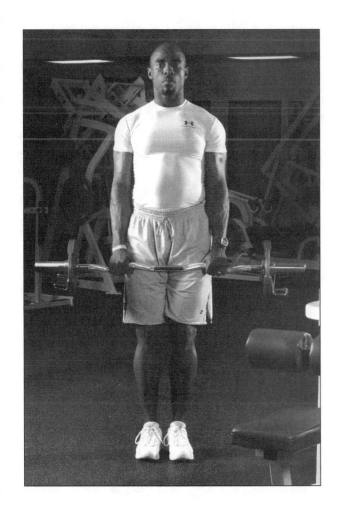 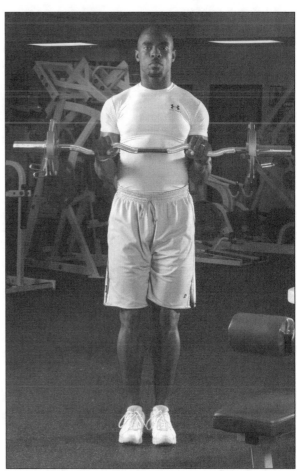

High Pulley One Arm Cable Curls

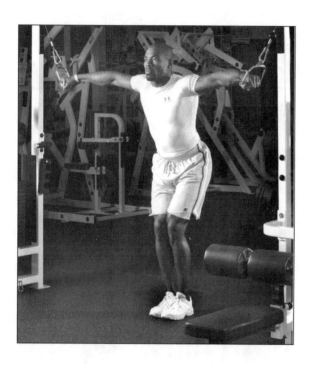 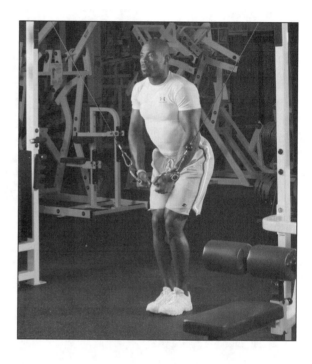

1 Stand between two high pulleys and grasp a handle in each hand. Your upper arms should be parallel to the floor, and the palms of your hands should face you.

2 Exhaling, flex your biceps and curl the handles towards you until they are next to your ears. Your upper arms should remain stationary, only your forearms moving. Hold for a second at the contracted position.

3 Slowly bring back the arms to the starting position.

Variations: If only one pulley is available, you can perform one arm at a time, or with a bar or E-Z attachment. With a bar, you face the pulley, with upper arms still parallel to the floor, and the bar is curled to almost touching your forehead.

Dumbbell Curls

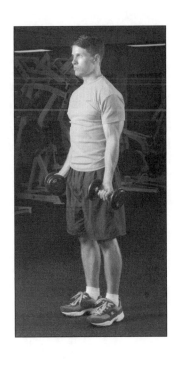 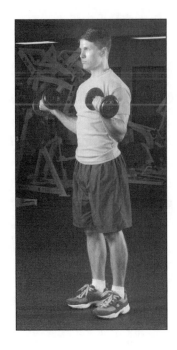

❶ Stand with a dumbbell in each hand held down near your thighs. Your elbows should be close to the torso, and the palms of your hands should face forward.

❷ Holding the upper arm stationary and exhale as you curl the weights up, contracting the biceps. Only your forearms should move. Continue the movement until the dumbbells are at shoulder height. Hold this position for a second.

❸ Inhale and slowly bring the dumbbells back to the starting position.

Variations: Try performing this exercise sitting at a bench with or without back support, or by alternating arms. Another possibility is to begin with palms facing your body, and then rotating forward as the curl progresses.

E-Z Reverse Preacher Curls

1 This exercise requires a preacher bench and an E-Z bar. Have your spotter hand you the bar, or use the front bar rest. Grasp the E-Z curl bar at the wide outer handle with the palms of your hands facing down and slightly tilted downward due to the shape of the bar. Your thumb should be higher than your little finger. Position your upper arms and chest against the preacher bench pad and hold the E-Z curl bar at shoulder length.

2 As you inhale, slowly lower the bar until your upper arm is extended and the biceps is fully stretched.

3 Exhale and use the biceps to curl the weight up until your biceps is fully contracted and the bar is at shoulder height.

Variations: Try using a low pulley with an E-Z bar attachment instead of an E-Z bar. You will need to position the bench in front of the pulley, and may also use a closer grip. You can use a straight bar as well; just remember that straight bars place more stress on the wrist joint.

E-Z Reverse Preacher Curls

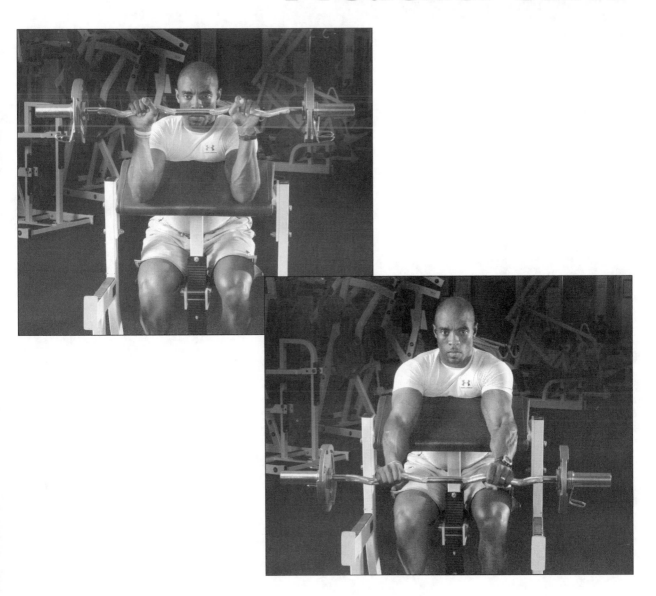

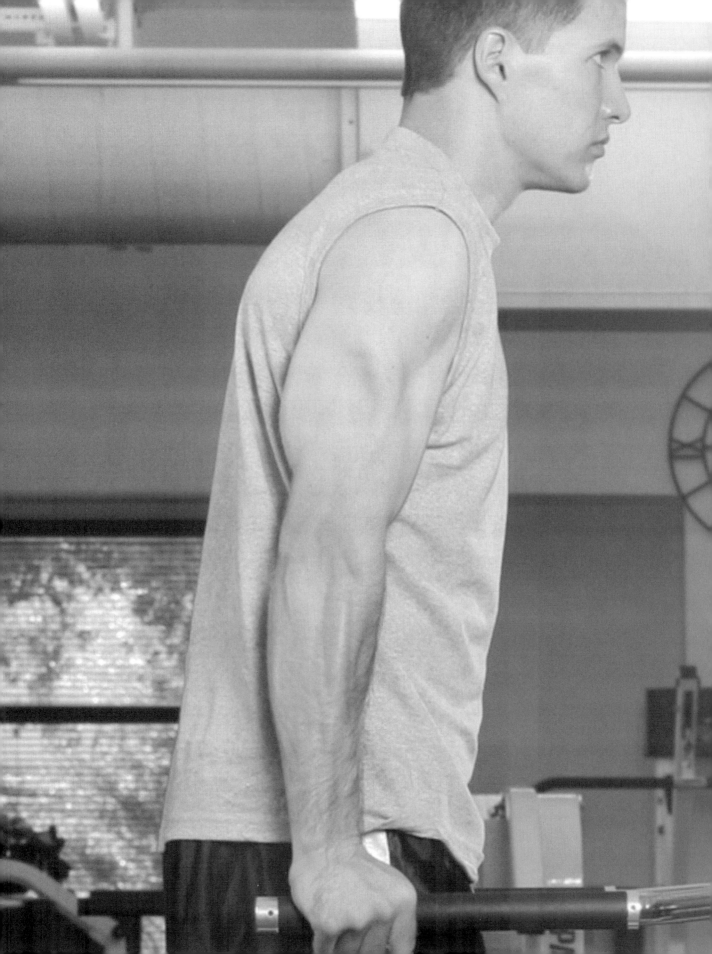

CHAPTER 11
Triceps Exercises

BASIC EXERCISES

Close Grip Bench Press

Triceps Dips

ISOLATION EXERCISES

Overhead Dumbbell
    Triceps Extensions

Lying Triceps Extensions

Triceps Kickbacks

Triceps Pushdowns

ALTERNATIVE EXERCISES

Bench Dips (Basic)

Fixed Bar Bodyweight
    Triceps Extensions (Isolation)

In this chapter we will cover the execution of all the triceps exercises presented in the routines of this program.

The triceps, while not as popular as the biceps, comprises two-thirds of your arm size, so if you want big arms you'd better work as hard on the triceps as you do on the biceps. The triceps are located on the backs of the upper arms, opposite to the biceps, and consist of three heads also originating at the shoulder and inserting below the elbow. In order to have a powerful-looking triceps, you need to develop all three heads. In order of appearance we will now cover the exercises used on this program and at the end of the chapter I will cover some additional useful exercises that can be used as well in lieu of the ones in the routines above.

Close Grip Bench Press

1 Lie back on a flat bench. Using a close grip (around shoulder width), lift the bar from the rack and hold it straight over you with your arms locked. This will be your starting position.

2 As you breathe in, come down slowly until you feel the bar on your middle chest. Make sure that, as opposed to a regular bench press, you keep the elbows close to the torso at all times.

3 After a second pause, bring the bar back to the starting position as you breathe out and push the bar using your triceps muscles. Lock your arms in the contracted position, hold for a second and then start coming down slowly again (it should take at least twice as long to go down as to come up).

4 Repeat the movement for the prescribed number of repetitions.

5 When you are done, place the bar back in the rack.

Caution: If you are new at this exercise, it is advised that you use a spotter. If no spotter is available, then be conservative with the amount of weight used. Also, beware of letting the bar drift too far toward your feet. You want the bar to fall on your middle chest and nowhere else.

Variations: This exercise can also be performed with an e-z bar using the inner handle with dumbbells in which case the palms of the hands will be facing each other.

Close Grip Bench Press

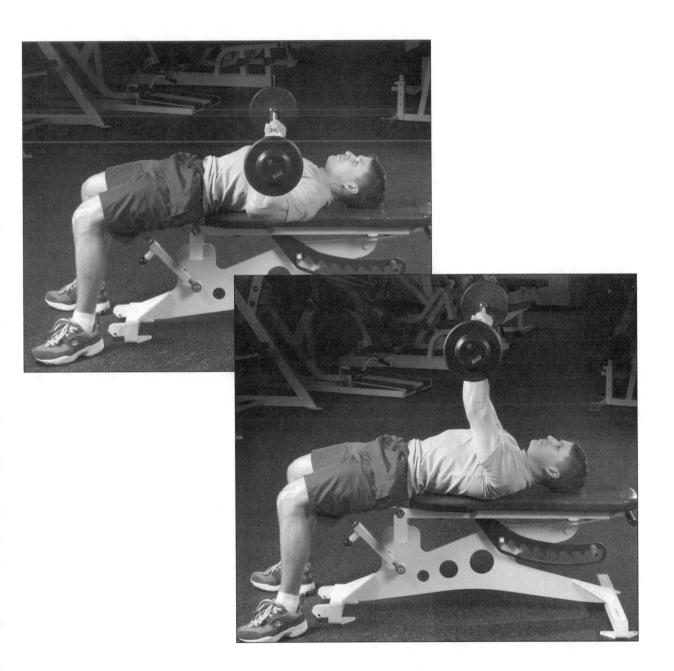

Triceps Dips

❶ For this exercise you will need access to parallel bars. To get yourself into the starting position, hold your body with locked, extended arms above the bars.

❷ While breathing in, lower yourself slowly with your torso as upright as possible and your elbows close to your body until there is a 90-degree angle (or slightly less) between the upper arm and the forearm.

❸ Push your torso up using your triceps to bring your body back to the starting position as you breathe out.

❹ Repeat the movement for the prescribed number of repetitions.

Variations: If you are new at this exercise and do not have the strength to perform it, use a dip assist machine if available. These machines use weight to help you push your body weight. Otherwise, a spotter holding your legs can help. If none of these two options are available, then substitute a barbell bench press, which is described later in this chapter. On the other hand, more advanced lifters can add weight to using a weight belt that allows the addition of weighted plates.

Triceps Dips

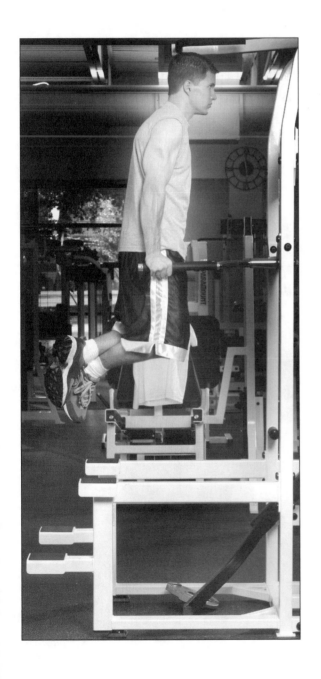 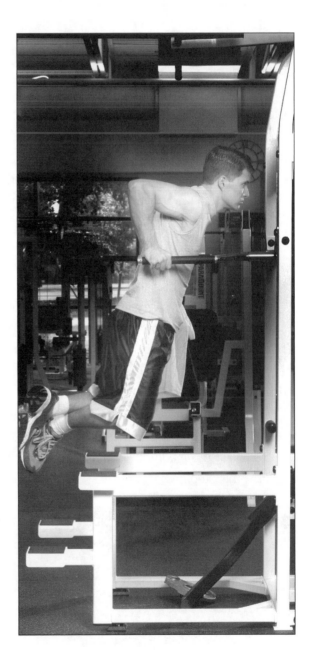

Overhead Dumbbell Triceps Extensions

❶ Seat down on a bench with back support and grasp a dumbbell with both hands and hold it overhead with arms fullly extended (note: a better way is to have somebody hand it to you, especially if it is very heavy). The resistance should be resting in the palms of your hands with your thumbs around it. The palm of the hand should be facing inward. This will be your starting position.

❷ Keeping your upper arms close to your head (elbows in) and perpendicular to the floor, lower the resistance in a semicircular motion behind your head until your forearms touch your biceps. The upper arms should remain stationary and only the forearms should move. Breathe in as you perform this step.

❸ Go back to the starting position by using the triceps to raise the dumbbell. Breathe out as you perform this step.

❹ Repeat for the recommended number of repetitions.

Variations: You can perform this exercise standing as well but this puts strain on your back, especially if you are using heavy dumbbells 95 lb or more. Another variation is to use an E-Z or straight bar instead, in which case you will be holding the bar from the inside (about 5 inches between your hands) with the palms facing forward (pronated grip). There is also a bar that has parallel bars inside (it's called a triceps blaster) and this can also be used for this exercise. Finally, a low pulley cable with a rope attachment or bar (straight or E-Z) attachment at the end can be used for variety.

Overhead Dumbbell Triceps Extensions

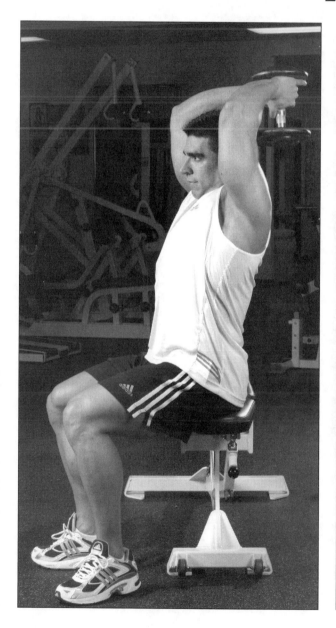 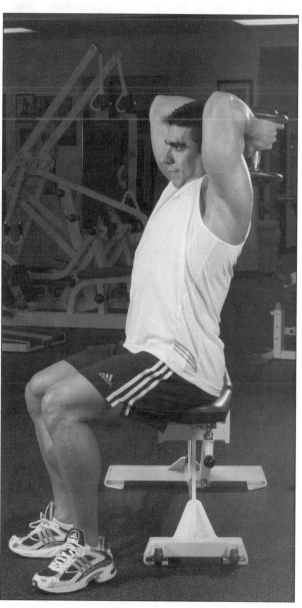

Lying Triceps Extensions

❶ Lie on a flat bench with either an E-Z bar (my preference) or a straight bar placed on the bench behind your head and your feet on the floor.

❷ Grab the bar behind you, using a medium overhand (pronated) grip, and raise the bar in front of you with arms fully extended. The arms should be perpendicular to the torso and the floor. The elbows should be tucked in. This is the starting position.

❸ As you breathe in, slowly lower the weight until the bar lightly touches your forehead while keeping the upper arms and elbows stationary.

❹ At that point, use the triceps to bring the weight back up to the starting position as you breathe out.

❺ Repeat for the recommended number of repetitions.

Caution: This is an exercise with which you need to be very careful with the weight selected and the form used. Too much weight and sloppy form and you could be looking at a head injury. Not to scare you off but the gym name of this exercise is "skull crushers." So please remember to be safe. Also, if you suffer from elbow problems this exercise might be too harsh on your elbows so you may need to look for a substitute such as a close-grip bench press.

Variations: There are a few variations of this exercise. You can perform it on a decline bench as opposed to a flat bench. You can also perform it using dumbbells in which case the palms of the hands will be facing each other as opposed to facing forward. Also, you can try to do it using a reverse grip (palms facing you) but this variation seems to strain my wrists.

Lying Triceps Extensions

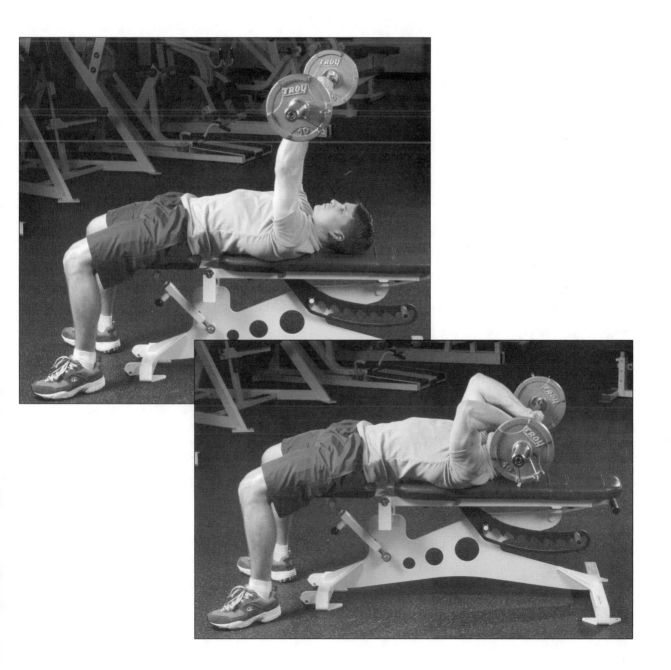

Triceps Kickbacks

❶ With a dumbbell in each hand, palms facing your torso, bend your knees slightly and bring your torso forward by bending at the waist, while keeping the back straight until it is almost parallel to the floor. Make sure that you keep the head up. The upper arms should be close to the torso and parallel to the floor while the forearms are pointing towards the floor as the hands hold the weights. There should be a 90-degree angle between the forearms and the upper arm. This is your starting position.

❷ Keeping the upper arms stationary, use the triceps to lift the weights as you exhale, until the forearms are parallel to the floor and the whole arms are extended. As in many other arm exercises, only the forearm moves.

❸ After a second contraction at the top, slowly lower the dumbbells back to their starting position as you inhale.

❹ Repeat the movement for the prescribed number of repetitions.

Variations: This exercise can also be executed one arm at a time much as the one-arm rows are performed. Also, if you like the one-arm variety, you can use a low pulley handle instead of a dumbbell for better peak contraction. In this case, the palms should be facing forward (supinated grip) as opposed toward the torso (neutral grip).

Triceps Kickbacks

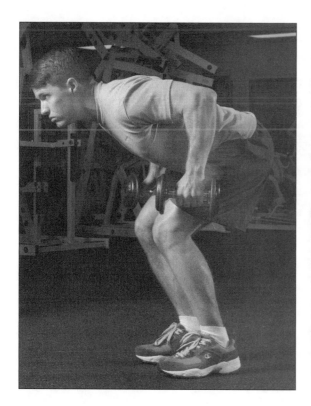 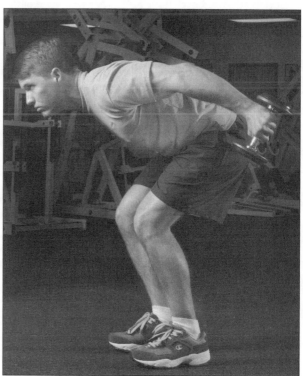

Triceps Pushdowns

1 Attach a straight bar to a high pulley and grab with an overhand grip (palms facing down) at shoulder width. Standing upright with the torso straight and a very small inclination forward, bring the upper arms close to your body and perpendicular to the floor. The forearms should be pointing up towards the pulley as they hold the bar. This is your starting position.

2 Using the triceps, bring the bar down until it touches the fronts of your thighs and the arms are fully extended perpendicular to the floor. The upper arms should always remain stationary next to your torso and only the forearms should move. Exhale as you perform this movement.

3 After a second hold at the contracted position, bring the bar slowly up to the starting point. Breathe in as you perform this step.

4 Repeat for the recommended number of repetitions.

Variations: There are many variations to this movement. For instance, you can use an e-z attachment as well as a V-angled bar that allows the thumb to be higher than the little finger. Also, you can attach a rope to the pulley as well as using a reverse grip on the bar exercises.

Triceps Pushdowns

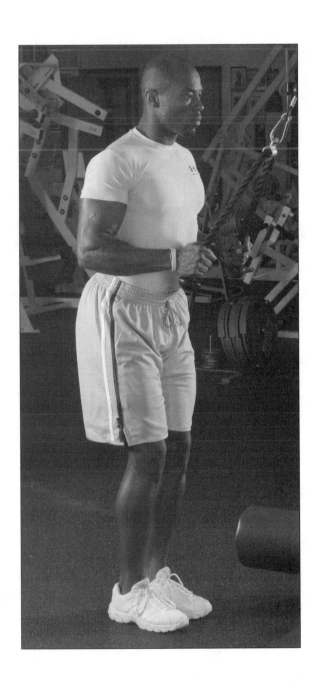 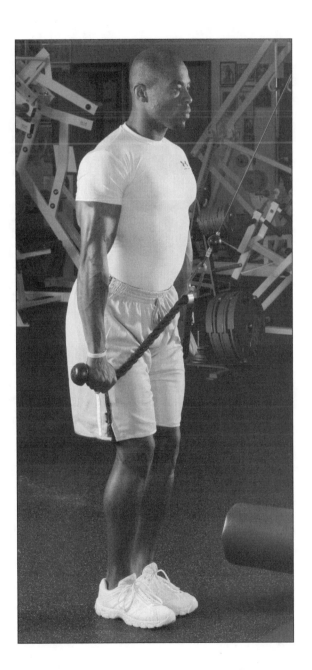

Bench Dips

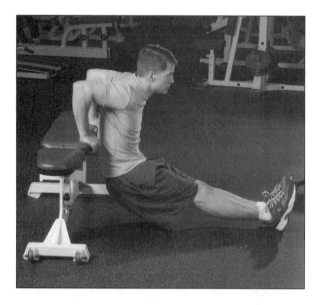 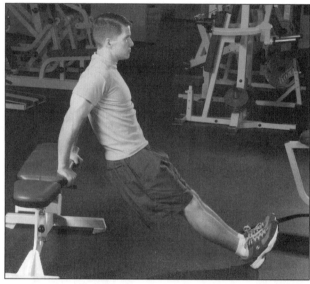

❶ Place a bench behind your back perpendicular to your body. Hold on to the edge with your hands fully extended, shoulder width apart. Your legs are extended forward, perpendicular to your torso.

❷ Inhale and slowly lower your body by bending at the elbows. Keep the elbows as close to the body as possible throughout the movement. Forearms should always be perpendicular with the floor.

❸ Using your triceps to lift your torso back to the starting position.

Variations: To make this more challenging, place your legs on top of another flat bench in front of you, or have your partner place plates on your lap.

Fixed Bar Bodyweight Triceps Extensions

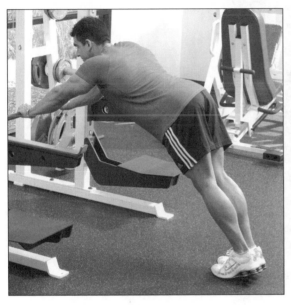
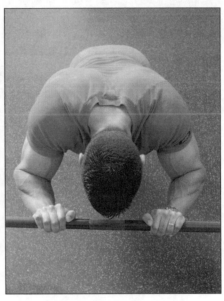

1 Fix a horizontal bar in front of at waist height. Do this by using the bar of a Smith machine or a regular Olympic bar placed at the end of a squat rack with adjustable pins.

2 Grasp the bar at shoulder width with an overhand grip (pronated). Your arms should extend forward at an angle of about 50 degrees from the head to the arms. Keep the rest of the torso straight but slanted forward so your arms are holding your weight and your legs are behind you as in a modified push-up position.

3 Keep your upper arms stationary and elbows in. Bend at the elbows and lower your body, inhaling, until your forehead lightly touches the bar.

4 Use your triceps to press against the bar, then exhale while bringing your torso back to the starting position.

Caution: This is a very advanced exercise that can only be performed by trainees with strength and gym experience.

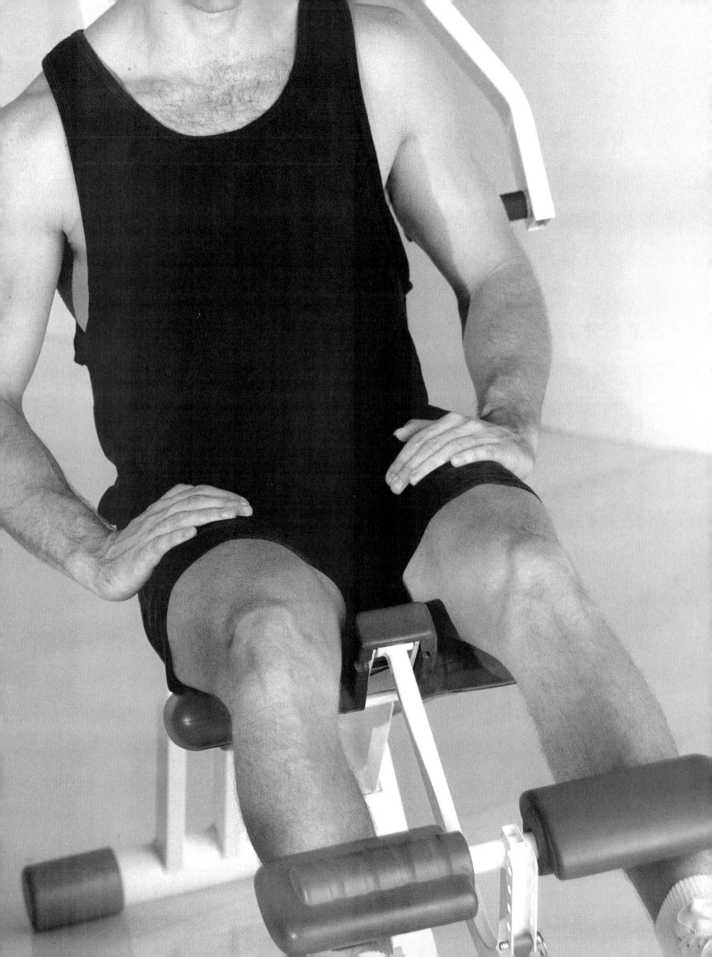

CHAPTER 12
Quadriceps Exercises

BASIC EXERCISES

Squats

Quadriceps Leg Press

ISOLATION EXERCISES

Leg Extensions

Sissy Squats

ALTERNATIVE EXERCISES

Hack Squats (Basic)

Dumbbell Lunges (Basic)

Front Squats (Basic)

In this chapter we will cover the execution of all the quadriceps exercises presented in the routines of this program.

The quadriceps are most often not worked hard enough by male bodybuilders. For some reason, most tend to concentrate more on the upper body than the lower body. However, nothing could be more of a mistake, especially if bodybuilding competition is a future goal. Even if competing is not on your mind, a big upper body supported by pencil-thin legs is not very aesthetically pleasing.

The quadriceps, just like the triceps in the upper arm, comprises most of the upper leg size. It is composed of four muscle heads located in the front of the leg whose main function is to push. In order to have a powerful-looking quadriceps, all four muscle heads need to be developed separately. This is done by using a variety of exercises and foot stances in order to emphasize a particular head at any given time. The following discussion talks about the different foot stances and their role in quadriceps development.

Foot Stances and Quadriceps Development

There are three main stances that we need to be concerned with:

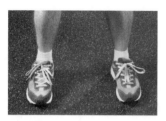

• **Shoulder-width stance** with toes pointed slightly out: This stance works best for stimulating overall thigh development.

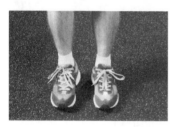

• **Close stance** with toes pointed straight ahead: This stance works best for stimulating growth of the outer quad, better known as the vastus lateralis. Note: Next time you watch the Olympics check out the vastus lateralis development of speed skaters; due to the nature of their sport, they have these muscles well developed.

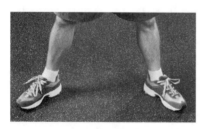

• **Wide stance** with toes pointed out at least 45 degrees: This stance targets both the vastus medialis, which is the inside head of the quadriceps near the knee, and the inner thigh or adductor muscles.

It is important to mention also that every time a quadriceps exercise is performed, it is imperative to push mainly with the toes as that will emphasize quadriceps recruitment.

For leg extension movements there are also three foot positions that can be used:

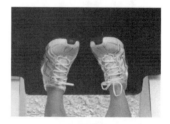

• **Toes straight:** Good for overall development.

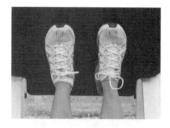

• **Toes in:** Good for maximizing outer quad (vastus lateralis) stimulation.

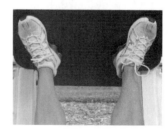

• **Toes out:** Good for maximizing inner quad (vastus medialis) stimulation.

Having said this, we will now cover in order of appearance the exercises used on this program and at the end of the chapter I will cover some additional useful exercises that can be used as well in lieu of the ones in the routines above.

Squats

FOOT STANCE: All stances

1 This exercise is best performed inside a squat rack for safety purposes. To begin, first set the bar on a rack that best matches your height. Once the correct height is chosen and the bar is loaded, step under the bar and place the back of your shoulders (slightly below the neck) across it.

2 Hold on to the bar using both arms at each side and lift it off the rack by first pushing with your legs and at the same time straightening your torso.

3 Step away from the rack and position your legs using a shoulder-width medium stance with the toes slightly pointed out. Keep your head up at all times as looking down will get you off balance, and also maintain a straight back. This will be your starting position. (Note: For the purposes of this discussion we will use the medium stance described above which targets overall development; however, you can choose any of the three stances).

4 Begin to slowly lower the bar by bending the knees as you maintain a straight posture with the head up. Continue down until the angle between the upper leg and the calves becomes slightly less than 90 degrees (which is the point at which the upper legs are below parallel to the floor). Inhale as you perform this portion of the movement. (Note: If you perform the exercise correctly, the fronts of the knees should make an imaginary straight line with the toes that is perpendicular to the torso. If your knees are past that imaginary line (if they are past your toes) then you are placing undue stress on the knees and the exercise has been performed incorrectly.)

5 Begin to raise the bar as you exhale by pushing the floor mainly with your toes as you straighten the legs again and go back to the starting position.

6 Repeat for the recommended number of repetitions.

Caution: This is not an exercise to be taken lightly. If you have back problems, substitute the dumbbell squat variation or a leg press instead. If you have a healthy back, maintain perfect form and never slouch the back forward as this can cause back injury. Be cautious as well with the weight used; in case of doubt, use less weight rather than more. The squat is a very safe exercise but only if performed properly.

Squats

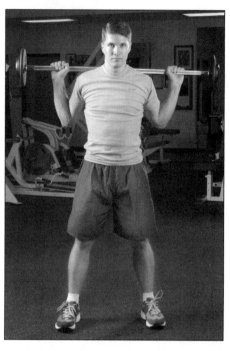
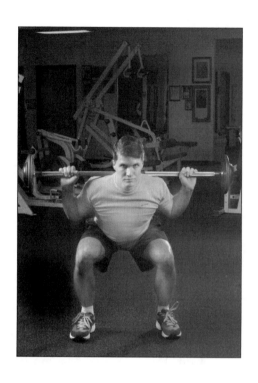

Variations: As previously mentioned, there are various stances that can be used depending on what you want to emphasize. You can also place a small block under the heels to improve balance.

Dumbbells can be used as well for resistance by holding them to your sides. The use of wrist wraps is a necessity due to the amount of weights used. I find this an excellent variation when my lower back begins to act up after many weeks of regular barbell squats. (Note: For wide stance dumbbell squats you will have to hold the dumbbells in between your legs

as opposed to both sides in order to be able to distance your legs sufficiently).

Another way to perform these is by using a weight belt and attaching weights to it in between the legs. This variation is referred to as weight belt squats. They need to be performed with the legs placed on two-well secured raised but separated platforms that allow the weights to go up and down in the middle. This exercise is an excellent choice for people with lower back problems. The issue, however, is finding platforms that meet the criteria. The only way I have been able to perform this is when I

Squats

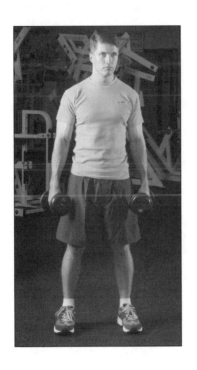 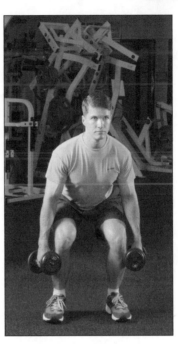

have two benches placed opposite to each other with spotting platforms that are facing each other. If you move the benches close enough you can execute the weight belt squats by using the spotting platform.

Finally, you can also perform squats in a Smith machine though I do not recommend this. The Smith machine allows you to execute the exercise while leaning, and hip flexor involvement is minimized, taking the hamstring out of the exercise. While this does take pressure off the lower back, hamstring involvement is a requirement to stabilize the kneecap. As a result, what is

created is a situation where destructive forces place a huge stress on the ACL (anterior cruciate ligament–a primary ligament in the knee capsule whose job is to provide knee stability) by pushing the kneecap forward. For this reason, I highly recommend against Smith machine use for squats and if you still insist on doing so, make sure it is a sporadic rather than frequent use.

Note: For the purposes of properly demonstrating the movement, a squat rack was not used.

Quadriceps Leg Press

FOOT STANCE: *All stances*

1 Using a leg press machine, sit down on the machine and place your legs on the platform directly in front of you at a medium (shoulder width) foot stance. (Note: For the purposes of this discussion we will use the medium stance described above which targets overall development; however, you can choose any of the three stances).

2 Lower the safety bars holding the weighted platform in place and press the platform all the way up until your legs are fully extended in front of you (Note: Do not lock your knees). Your torso and the legs should make a perfect 90-degree angle. This will be your starting position.

3 As you inhale, slowly lower the platform until your upper and lower legs make a 90-degree angle.

4 Pushing mainly with the toes and using the quadriceps, go back to the starting position as you exhale.

5 Repeat for the recommended number of repetitions and be sure to lock the safety pins properly once you are done. You do not want that platform falling on you fully loaded.

Caution: Call me extra careful but when I am done with a set I exit the machine by getting my legs out first to one side and then my body. I have seen cases where the safety locks have failed and the whole platform comes tumbling down. Luckily in none of the cases was anyone sitting on the machine but if somebody's legs had been inside the machine at the time a serious accident could have occurred. As a result, I exit the machine after every set.

Variations: All foot-stance variations described at the beginning of the chapter.

Quadriceps Leg Press

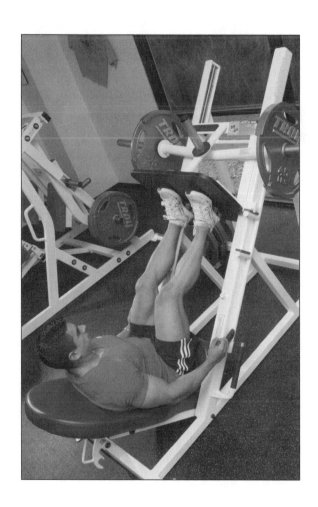
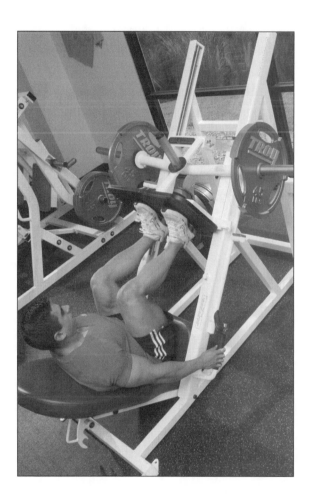

Leg Extensions

FOOT STANCE: *All foot positions*

❶ For this exercise you will need to use a leg extension machine. First choose your weight and sit on the machine with your legs under the pad (feet pointed forward) and the hands holding the sidebars. This will be your starting position. Note: You will need to adjust the pad so that it falls on top of your lower leg (just above your feet). Also, make sure that your legs form a 90-degree angle between the lower and upper leg. If the angle is less than 90 degrees, that means the knee is over the toes, which creates undue stress at the knee joint. If the machine is designed that way, either look for another machine or just make sure that when you start executing the exercise you stop going down once you hit the 90-degree angle.

❷ Using your quadriceps, extend your legs to the maximum as you exhale. Ensure that the rest of the body remains stationary on the seat. Pause a second on the contracted position.

❸ Slowly lower the weight to the original position as you inhale, ensuring that you do not go past the 90-degree angle limit.

❹ Repeat for the recommended number of times.

Variations: As mentioned at the beginning of this chapter, you can use various foot positions in order to maximize stimulation of certain thigh areas. Also, you can perform the movement unilaterally (one leg at a time).

Notes: During the leg extensions, pause for a second at the top of the contraction and then lower yourself slowly.

Leg Extensions

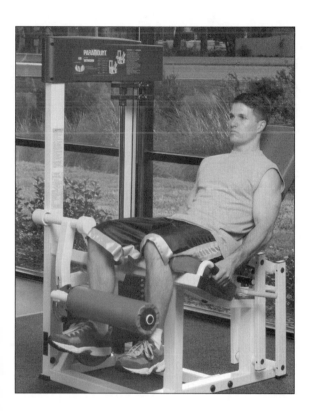 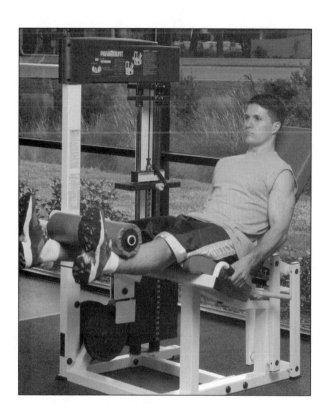

Sissy Squats

❶ Standing upright, with feet at shoulder width and heels raised, hold onto a stationary object for support (I typically use one of the beams of a squat rack). This is your starting position.

❷ As you use one arm to hold yourself (or both if in the middle of the squat rack), bend at the knees and slowly lower your torso toward the ground by bringing your pelvis and knees forward. Inhale as you go down and stop when your buttocks almost touch your heels. Hold the stretch position for a second.

❸ After your one second hold, use your thigh muscles to bring your torso back up to the starting position. Exhale as you move up.

❹ Repeat for the recommended number of times.

Caution: This exercise is to be avoided if you suffer from knee problems as it can stress the knee. Also, make sure that there is nothing behind you so if you lose your balance and fall that way nothing will hit you on the head causing an injury.

Variations: If you are new to this exercise, you can start by using two arms (so you'll need the two beams of the squat rack in front of you to hold yourself). As you become more advanced, just use one arm. Once that becomes easy you can use the opposite arm to hold a plate on top of your chest. There are no foot stance variations.

Notes: Ensure that your hamstrings touch the calves at the bottom of the movement to emphasize the stretch portion.

Sissy Squats

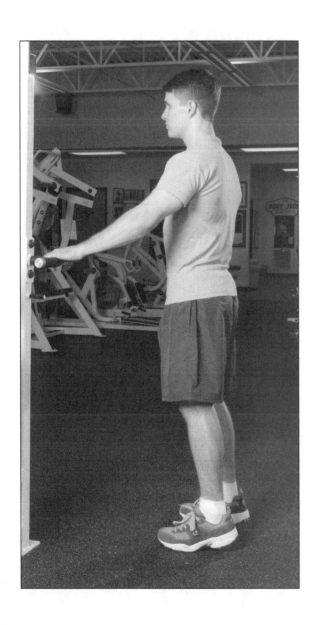 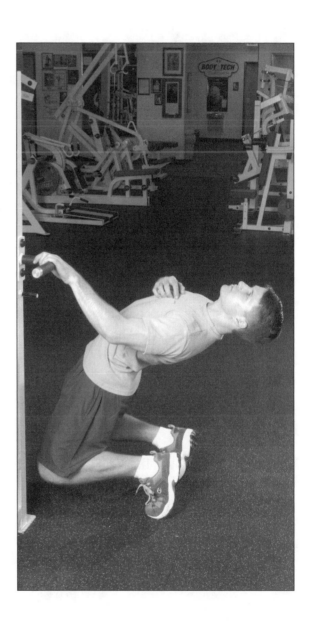

Hack Squats

❶ Place the back of your torso against the back pad of the Hack Squat machine and hook your shoulder under the shoulder pad provided. Position your legs in the platform using a shoulder width stance, toes slightly pointed out. Make sure to keep your head up at all times and keep your back against the pad. (You can move your back, but the pad stays in one place.) Place your arms on the side handles of the machine and disengage the safety bars, and straighten your legs without locking your knees.

❷ Begin to slowly lower the unit by bending your knees. Continue down, inhaling as you do so, until your upper legs are slightly below parallel to the floor. The fronts of the knees should make an imaginary straight line with the toes that is perpendicular to the torso.

❸ Begin to raise the unit as you exhale by pushing the floor with your toes, straightening your legs, and returning to the starting position.

Variations: Try this with many different foot positions.

Hack Squats

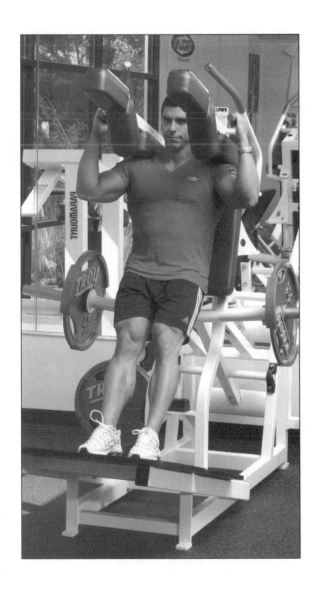 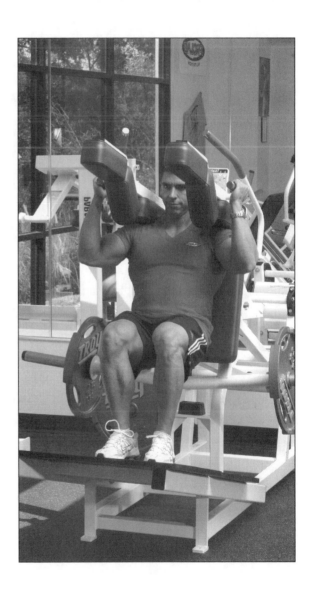

Dumbbell Lunges

QUADRICEPS EMPHASIS: Toe press

1 Stand with your torso upright holding two dumbbells in your hands by your sides.

2 While inhaling, take a 2-foot step with your right leg, keeping your left leg stationary, and lower your upper body. Keep your torso upright and balanced as you descend. Do not allow your knee to move beyond your toes, as this will put undue stress on the knee joint. Your front shin should be perpendicular to the ground.

3 Push up using your toes and, exhaling, return to the starting position.

4 Repeat the movement for the recommended number of repetitions with one leg and then switch the leading leg.

Caution: This requires a great deal of balance. If you suffer from balance problems, use your own body weight while holding on to a fixed object, and do not attempt to use a barbell on your back.

Variations: Try alternating legs, or static lunges, which require you to start leading with your leg already placed forward. In this case, you just go up and down from the starting position, then switch legs and repeat. For a challenge, try walking lunges which require you to walk across the room by lunging, bringing the lagging leg forward after the lunge to continue moving ahead. Lunges use either dumbbells or a barbell placed on the back.

Dumbbell Lunges

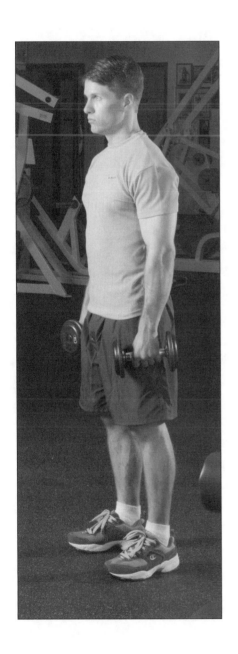
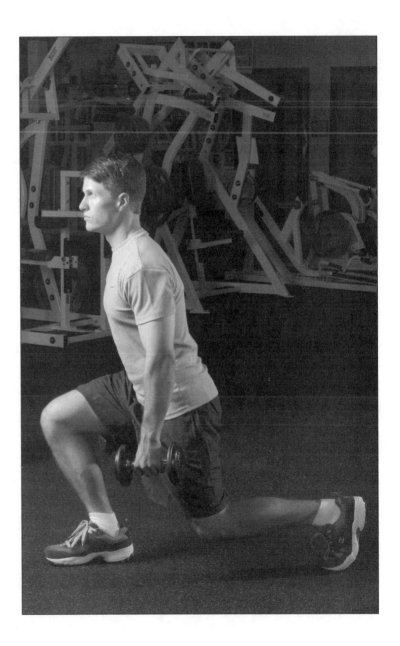

Front Squats

FOOT STANCE: *All stances*

1 This exercise is best performed inside a squat rack for safety purposes. To begin, first set the bar on a rack that best matches your height. Bring your arms up under the bar, keeping elbows high and your upper arm slightly above parallel to the floor. Rest the bar on top of the deltoids and cross your arms while grasping the bar for total control.

2 Lift the bar off the rack by first pushing with your legs and at the same time straightening your torso.

3 Step away from the rack and position your legs using a shoulder width stance, your toes slightly pointed out. Your head should be up at all times to maintain a straight back. This will be your starting position.

4 Inhale and slowly bend your knees, continuing down until your upper legs are slightly below parallel to the floor. The fronts of your knees should not be past your toes, or you are placing undue stress on the knee and performing the exercise incorrectly.

5 Raise the bar again, exhaling and pushing the floor with your toes to straighten your legs and return to the starting position.

Caution: If you have back problems, substitute the dumbbell squat variation or a leg press instead. If you have a healthy back, maintain perfect form and never slouch forward as this can cause injury. Use less weight rather than more if you are new to this exercise. The squat is very safe, but only if performed properly, and this version is better suited to advanced athletes.

Variations: There are various stances that can be used depending on what muscle group you wish to emphasize. You can also place a small block under the heels to improve balance.

Note: For the purposes of properly demonstrating the movement, a squat rack was not used.

Front Squats

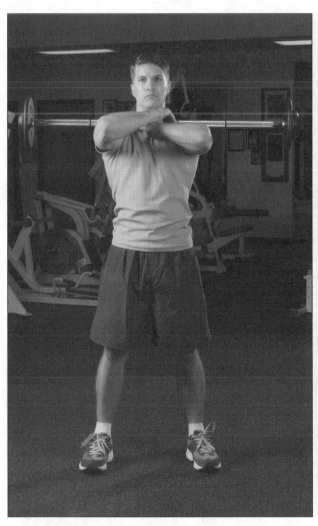 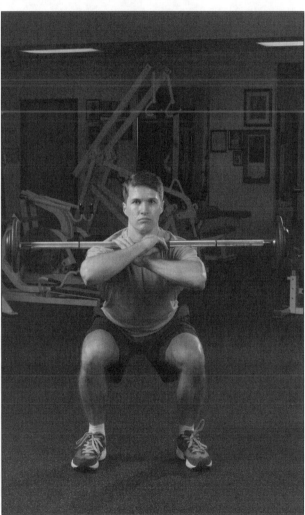

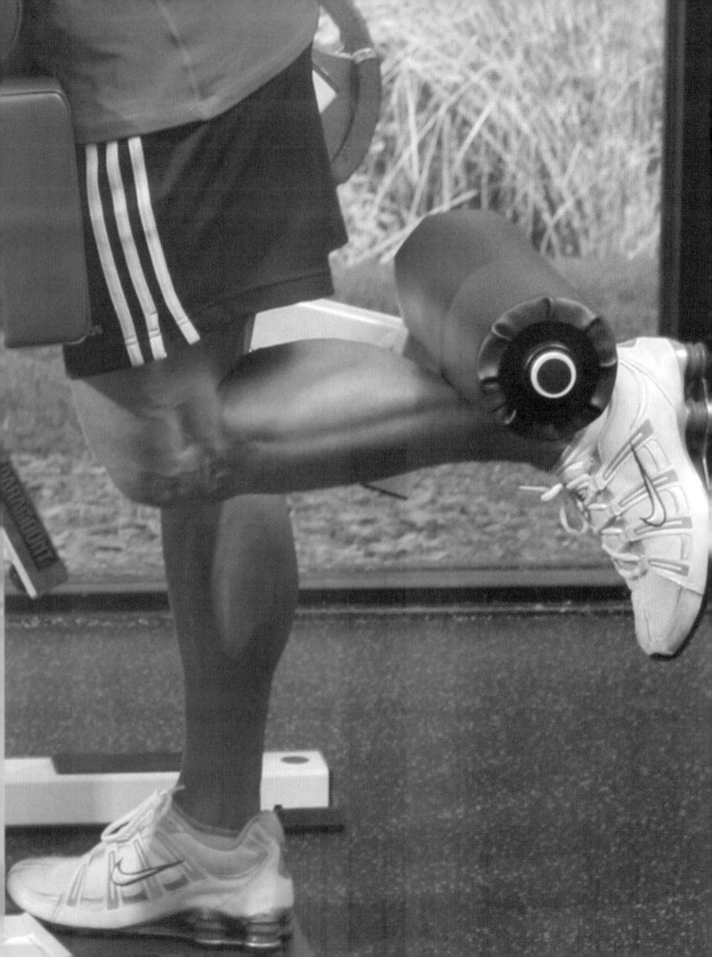

CHAPTER 13
Hamstring Exercises

BASIC EXERCISES

Dumbbell Lunges

Hamstrings Leg Press

Dumbbell Stiff-Legged Deadlifts

Barbell Stiff-Legged Deadlifts

ISOLATION EXERCISES

Lying Leg Curls

ALTERNATIVE EXERCISES

Inner Thigh/
    Hamstring Squats (Basic)

Step-Ups (Basic)

Standing Leg Curls (Isolation)

Seated Leg Curls (Isolation)

Glute-Ham Raises (Isolation)

In this chapter we will cover the execution of all the hamstring exercises presented in the routines of this program.

The hamstrings are even more neglected than the quadriceps. While working out the quadriceps does provide indirect hamstring stimulation at the bottom of compound movements like squats and leg presses, in order to have nice hamstrings this muscle needs to be paid the same amount of attention that the quadriceps gets. The hamstrings are analogous to the biceps on the upper arm. Their function is to flex the knee and extend the hip. As a result, in order to work this muscle thoroughly, both knee flexion (as in a leg curl) and hip extension (as in a stiff-legged dead lift) need to be included in your program.

The hamstrings are composed of three muscle heads located in the back of the leg (the biceps femoris, semitendinosus, and semimembranosus) whose main function is to pull the lower leg towards the glutes and also to extend the hip. In order to have powerful-looking hamstrings, both the knee flexion muscles and the hip extension muscles need to be stimulated.

Foot Stances and Hamstrings Development

For the hamstring leg press or inner thigh squat movement, there is only one main stance that we need to be concerned with:

Wide stance with toes pointed out at least 45 degrees. Force is exerted by pressing with the heel. This stance targets the glute and the part of the hamstring that attaches there.

It is important to mention also that every time a hamstring pressing type of exercise is performed, it is imperative to push mainly with the heels as that will emphasize hamstring/glute recruitment.

For leg curl type movements there are three foot positions that can be used:

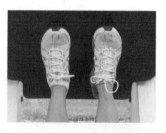

1. **Toes Straight:** Good for overall development.

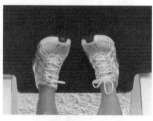

2. **Toes In:** Good for maximizing inner hamstring (semitendinosus and semimembranosus) head stimulation.

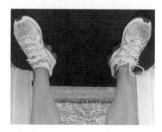

3. **Toes Out:** Good for maximizing outer hamstring (biceps femoris) head stimulation.

Having said this, we will now cover in order of appearance the exercises used on this program and at the end of the chapter I will cover some additional useful exercises that can be used as well in lieu of the ones in the routines above.

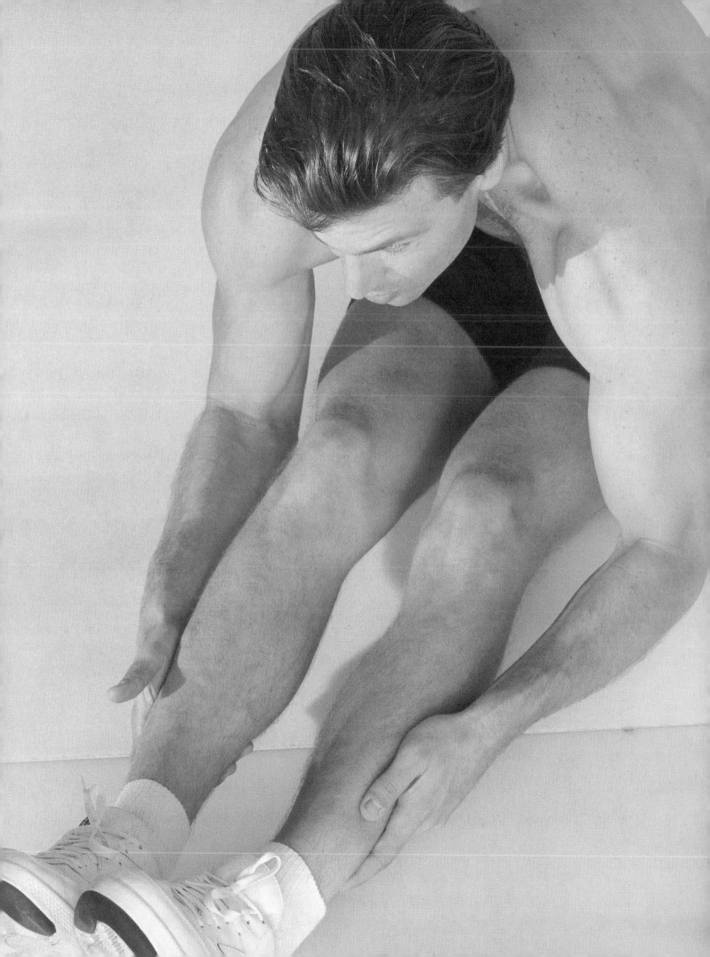

Dumbbell Lunges

HAMSTRING EMPHASIS: *Heel Press*

1 Stand with your torso upright holding two dumbbells in your hands by your sides. This will be your starting position.

2 Step forward with your right leg about 2 feet or so from the foot being left stationary behind and lower your upper body, while keeping the torso upright and maintaining balance. Inhale as you go down. Note: As in the other exercises, do not allow your knee to go forward beyond your toes as you come down, as this will put undue stress on the knee joint. Make sure that you keep your front shin perpendicular to the ground.

3 Using mainly your heel, push up and go back to the starting position as you exhale.

4 Repeat the movement for the recommended number of repetitions and then perform with the left leg.

Caution: This is a movement that requires a great deal of balance, so if you suffer from balance problems you may wish to either avoid it or just use your own body weight while holding on to a fixed object. Definitely never perform with a barbell on your back if you suffer from balance problems.

Variations: There are several ways to perform the exercise. One way is to alternate legs. For instance, do one repetition with the right, then the left, then the right and so on. The other way is to do what I call a static lunge where your start with one of your feet already forward. In this case, you just go up and down from the starting position until you are done with the recommended number of repetitions. Then you switch legs and do the same. A more challenging version is the walking lunges where you walk across the room by lunging. For walking lunges the leg being left back has to be brought forward after the lunging action has happened in order to continue moving ahead. This version is reserved for the most advanced athletes.

Lunges can be performed with dumbbells as described above or with a barbell on the back, though the barbell variety is better suited for advanced athletes who have mastered the exercise and no longer have balance problems.

Dumbbell Lunges

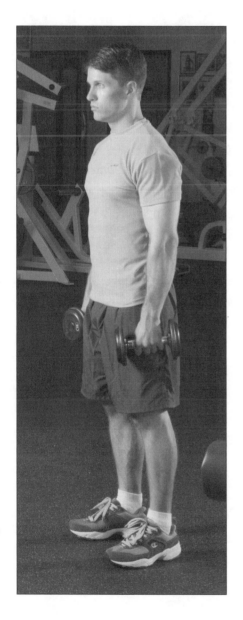
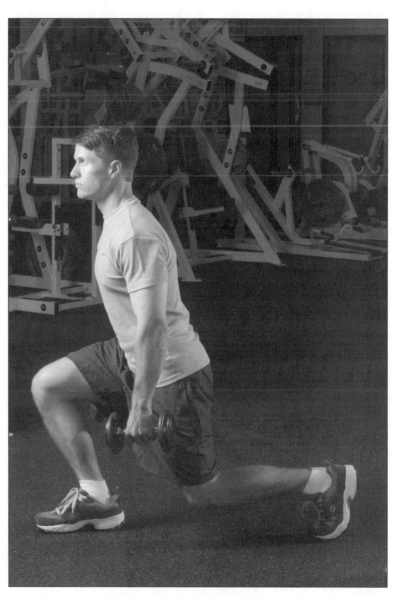

Hamstrings Leg Press

FOOT STANCE: *With feet high on platform and wide stance. Press with heel.*

❶ Using a leg press machine, sit down on the machine and place your legs high on the platform at a wide stance with toes pointed at least 45 degrees out.

❷ Lower the safety bars holding the weighted platform in place and press the platform all the way up until your legs are fully extended in front of you (Note: Do not lock your knees). Your torso and legs should make a perfect 90-degree angle. This will be your starting position.

❸ As you inhale, slowly lower the platform until your upper and lower legs bend past a 90-degree angle.

❹ Pushing mainly with the heels and using the glutes and hamstrings, go back to the starting position as you exhale.

❺ Repeat for the recommended number of repetitions and ensure to lock the safety pins properly once you are done. You do not want the platform falling on you fully loaded.

Caution: Call me extra careful but when I am done with a set I exit the machine by getting my legs out first to one side and then my body. I have seen cases where the safety locks have failed and the whole platform comes tumbling down. Luckily, in none of the cases was anyone sitting on the machine ,but if somebody's legs would have been inside the machine at the time a serious accident could have occurred. As a result, I exit the machine after every set.

Also, if you experience any knee pains during the exercise, you may wish to substitute a wide stance squat or a deadlift movement as this exercise could be hard on the knees.

Hamstrings Leg Press

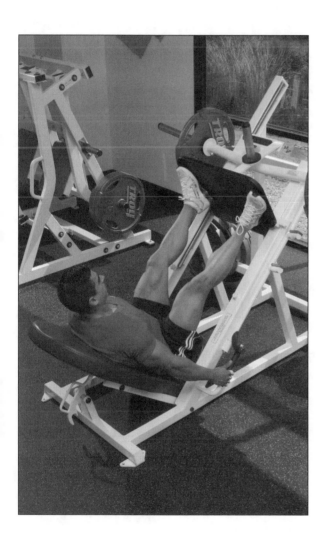
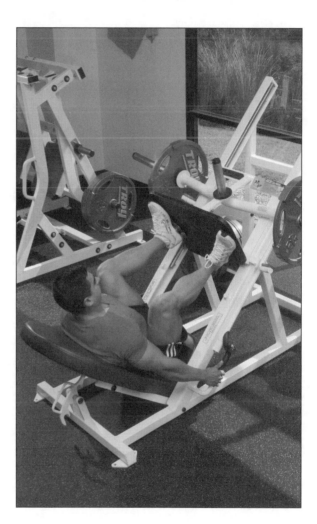

Dumbbell Stiff-Legged Deadlift

1 Grasp a couple of dumbbells and hold them by your sides.

2 Stand with your torso straight and a shoulder-width or narrower stance. The knees should be slightly bent. This is your starting position.

3 Keeping the knees stationary, lower the dumbbells to over the top of your feet by bending at the waist while keeping your back straight. Keep moving forward as if you were going to pick something from the floor until you feel a stretch on the hamstrings. Exhale as you perform this movement.

4 Start bringing your torso up straight again by extending your hips and waist until you are back at the starting position. Inhale as you perform this movement.

5 Repeat for the recommended number of repetitions.

Caution: This is not an exercise that is recommended for people with lower back problems. Also, it needs to be treated with the utmost respect, paying special care not to round the back forward as you move the torso down; the back should always be straight. Finally, jerking motions or using too much weight can injure your back.

Variations: The exercise can also be performed with a barbell as described below.

Notes: When on the stiff-legged deadlifts, go down slowly and deliberately to get a nice stretch, and return to a standing position in an equally slow manner. Be very careful with the execution of this exercise as bad form can cause a lower back injury.

Dumbbell Stiff-Legged Deadlift

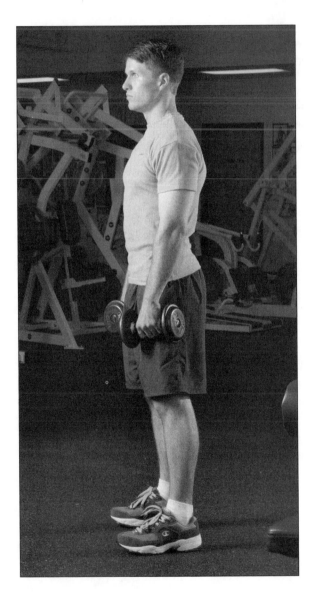

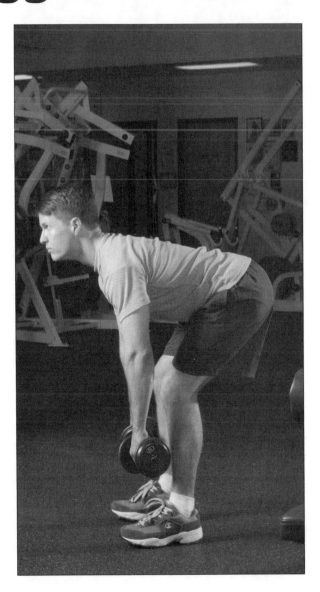

Barbell Stiff-Legged Deadlifts

1 Grasp a bar using an overhand grip (palms facing down). You may need some wrist wraps if using a significant amount of weight.

2 Stand with your torso straight and your legs spaced using a shoulder-width or narrower stance. The knees should be slightly bent. This is your starting position.

3 Keeping the knees stationary, lower the barbell to over the tops of your feet by bending at the waist while keeping your back straight. Keep moving forward as if you were going to pick something from the floor until you feel a stretch on the hamstrings. Exhale as you perform this movement.

4 Start bringing your torso up straight again by extending your hips and waist until you are back at the starting position. Inhale as you perform this movement.

5 Repeat for the recommended number of repetitions.

Caution: This is not an exercise that is recommended for people with lower back problems. Also, it needs to be treated with the utmost respect, taking special care not to round the back forward as you move the torso down; the back should always be straight. Finally, jerking motions or using too much weight can injure your back.

Variations: The exercise can also be performed with a dumbbell as described above.

Barbell Stiff-Legged Deadlifts

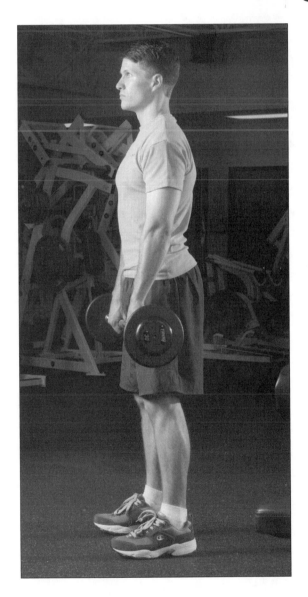 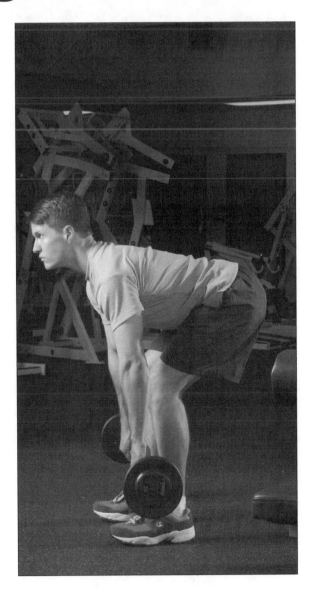

Lying Leg Curls

FOOT STANCE: *All stances*

1 Adjust the machine lever to fit your height and lie face down on the leg curl machine (preferably one where the pad is angled as opposed to flat since an angled position is more favorable to hamstrings recruitment) with the pad of the lever on the back of your legs just a few inches under the calves.

2 Keeping the torso flat on the bench, keep your legs fully stretched and grab the side handles of the machine. Position your toes straight (or use any of the other two stances). This will be your starting position.

3 As you exhale, curl your legs up as far as possible without lifting the upper legs from the pad. Once you hit the fully contracted position, hold it for a second.

4 As you inhale, bring the legs back to the initial position. Repeat for the recommended number of repetitions.

Cautions: Do not ever use so much weight on the exercise that you start swinging and jerking as you can risk both lower back injury and a hamstring tear.

Variations: Since you have three foot positions you have in reality three exercises. The movement can also be performed with a dumbbell held in between your feet (a partner needs to place it properly). This latter exercise, though, is only suitable for advanced trainees. Finally, it is also possible to use just one leg at a time for better isolation.

Lying Leg Curls

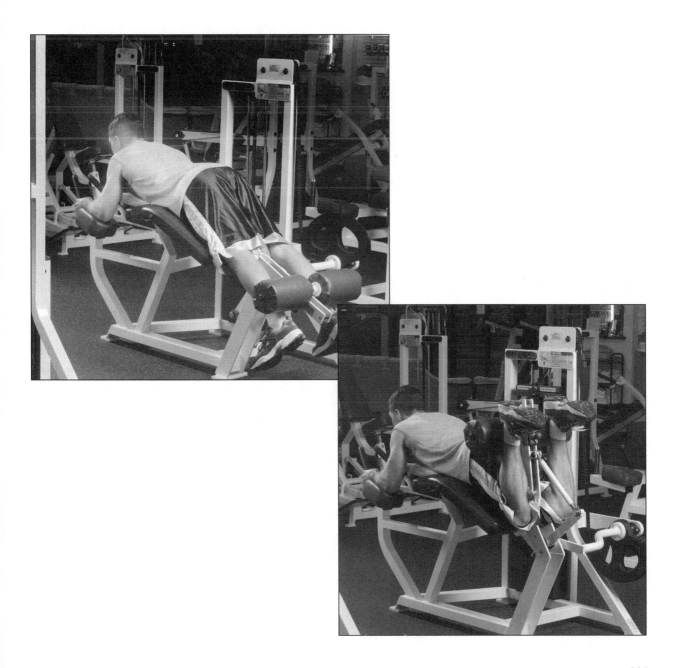

Inner Thigh/ Hamstring Squats

1 This exercise is best performed inside a squat rack for safety purposes. First set the bar on a rack that best matches your height. Then step under the bar and place the back of your shoulders (slightly below the neck) across it. Hold on to the bar using both arms at each side and lift it off the rack by first pushing with your legs and at the same time straightening your torso.

2 Step away from the rack and position your legs using a wide stance with the toes pointed out at 45-degree angles. Keep your head up at all times to maintain a straight back.

3 Inhaling, slowly bend at the knees, continuing down until the upper leg is slightly below parallel to the floor. If your knees are past your toes, then you are placing undue stress on the knee and the exercise has been performed incorrectly.

4 As you exhale, raise the bar by pushing at the floor with your heels as you straighten the legs again and go back to the starting position.

Caution: If you have back problems, substitute the dumbbell squat variation or a leg press. If you have a healthy back, maintain perfect form and never slouch the back forward. Be careful with the amount of weight used. The squat is a very safe exercise, but only if performed properly.

Variations: Dumbbells may be used for resistance by holding them between your legs. The use of wrist wraps is a necessity due to the amount of weights used. You may also use a weight belt between the legs and attach weights to it. This is called weight belt squats, and requires the legs to be placed on two well-secured raised but separated platforms that allow the weights to go up and down in the middle. You can also perform squats in a Smith machine, although this is not recommended because the Smith machine reduces stability by eliminating hamstring involvement, potentially leading to injury.

Note: For the purposes of properly demonstrating the movement, a squat rack was not used.

Inner Thigh/ Hamstring Squats

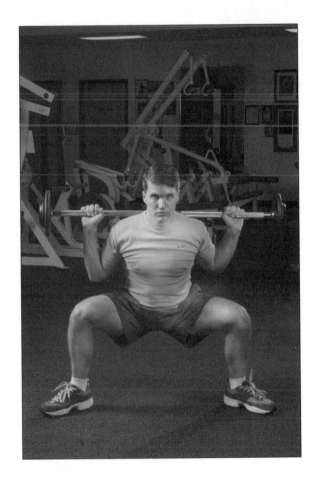 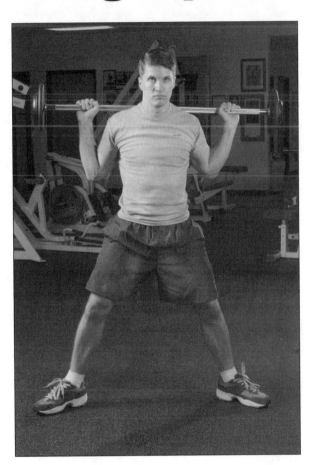

Step-Ups

1 Hold a pair of dumbbells at your sides and stand behind an elevated platform.

2 Place your right foot on the elevated platform. Step onto the platform by extending the hip and the knee of your right leg. Use the heel to lift the rest of your body up and place the foot of the left leg on the platform as well. Exhale as you push up.

3 Step down with the left leg by flexing the hip and knee of the right leg as you inhale. Return to the original standing position by placing the right foot next to the left foot in the initial position.

Variations: Just like lunges, this exercise can also be performed by alternating legs until all repetitions have been performed. To make this more difficult, a barbell can be used. To make this easier, stay with body weight only.

Step-Ups

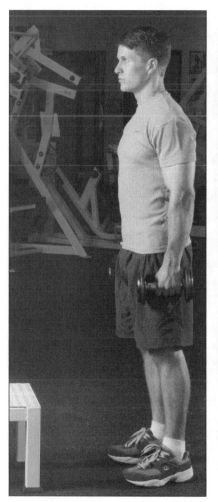
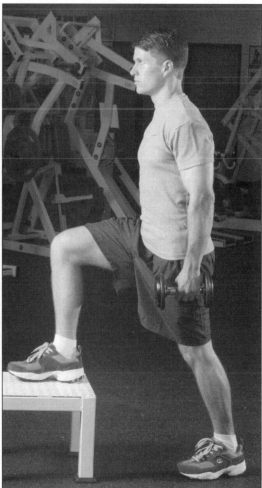
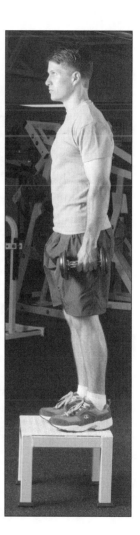

Standing Leg Curls

FOOT STANCE: All stances

1 Adjust the machine to fit your height. Lie with your torso bent slightly at the waist with the pad of the lever on the back of your right leg and the front of the right leg against the machine pad.

2 Keep your torso bent forward, ensure your leg is fully stretched, and grasp the side handles of the machine. Your toes should be straight.

3 As you exhale, curl your right leg up as far as possible without lifting the upper leg from the pad. Once you hit the fully contracted position, hold it for a second.

4 As you inhale, bring the legs back to the initial position. Repeat for the recommended number of repetitions. Switch legs when you are ready.

Cautions: Never use so much weight that you start using a swinging motion, as this can lead to a lower back injury and cause a hamstring tear.

Variations: Try this with another foot position. A dumbbell can also be held in between your feet, placed properly by your spotter, as your upper body hangs from a chin-up bar. This requires wrist wraps and is only suitable for advanced trainees. It is also possible to just use one leg at a time for better isolation.

Standing Leg Curls

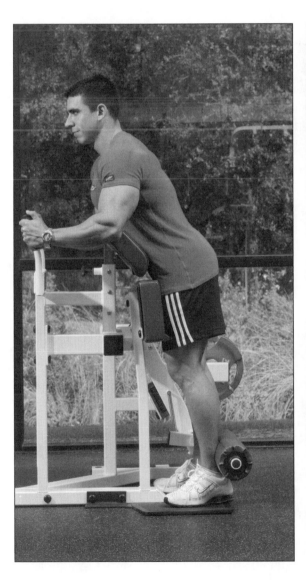 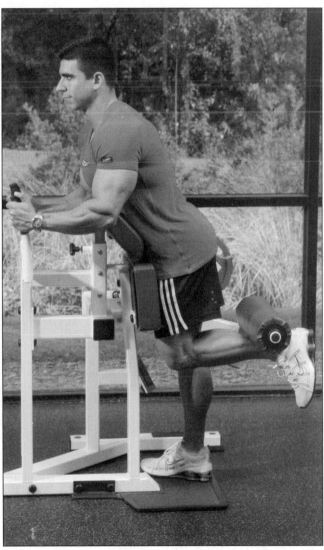

Seated Leg Curls

FOOT STANCE: *All stances*

1 Adjust the machine lever to fit your height and sit on the machine with your back against the back support pad. Place the back of your lower leg on top of the padded lever and secure the lap pad against your thighs, just above the knees. Grasp the side handles on the machine as you point your toes straight and ensure that the legs are fully straight right in front of you.

2 As you exhale, pull the machine lever as far as possible to the back of your thighs by flexing at the knees. Keep your torso stationary at all times. Hold the contracted position for a second.

3 Inhale and slowly return to the starting position.

Cautions: Never use so much weight that you swing, as this leads to lower back injury and hamstring tears.

Variations: Try this with another foot position.

Seated Leg Curls

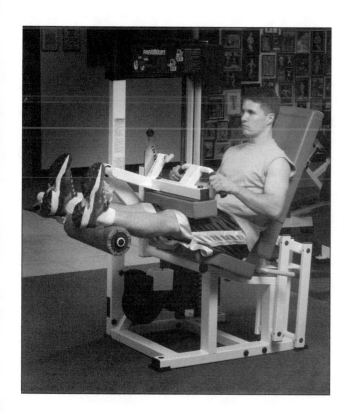
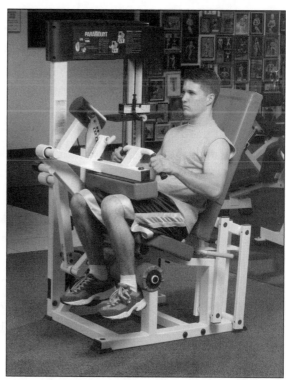

Glute-Ham Raises

1 You will need access to the seat of a pulldown machine. Adjust the padded supports of the pulldown machine and kneel upright in the seat of the apparatus.

2 Position your knees on top of the seat of the machine so you face away, with your ankles between the padded supports, and feet below the platform where typically the thighs are held in place. There should be a 90-degree angle created by the upper leg and lower leg.

3 Bring your torso forward by thrusting your hips forward, straightening your knees slightly. As the torso comes down you should inhale and not allow for any bending at the waist area; only your knees should be bending.

4 As you exhale, pull your body upright by flexing at the knees until you are back at the original position.

Caution: If you are a beginner, a spotter's presence is imperative for this advanced exercise. This may be hard on the lower back.

Variations: To make this easier, use a pole or a training partner to assist in getting to the upright position. To make this more difficult, weight can be added by holding a plate on the chest.

Glute-Ham Raises

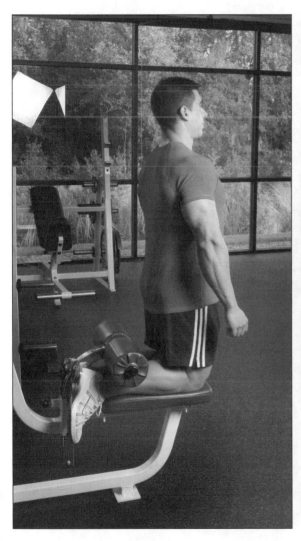 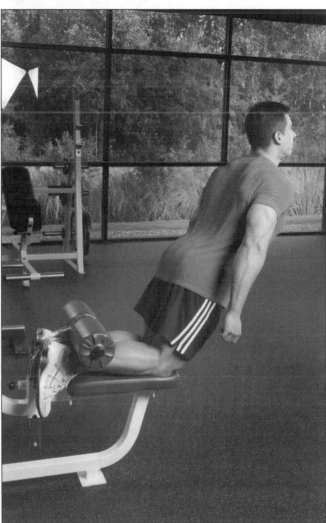

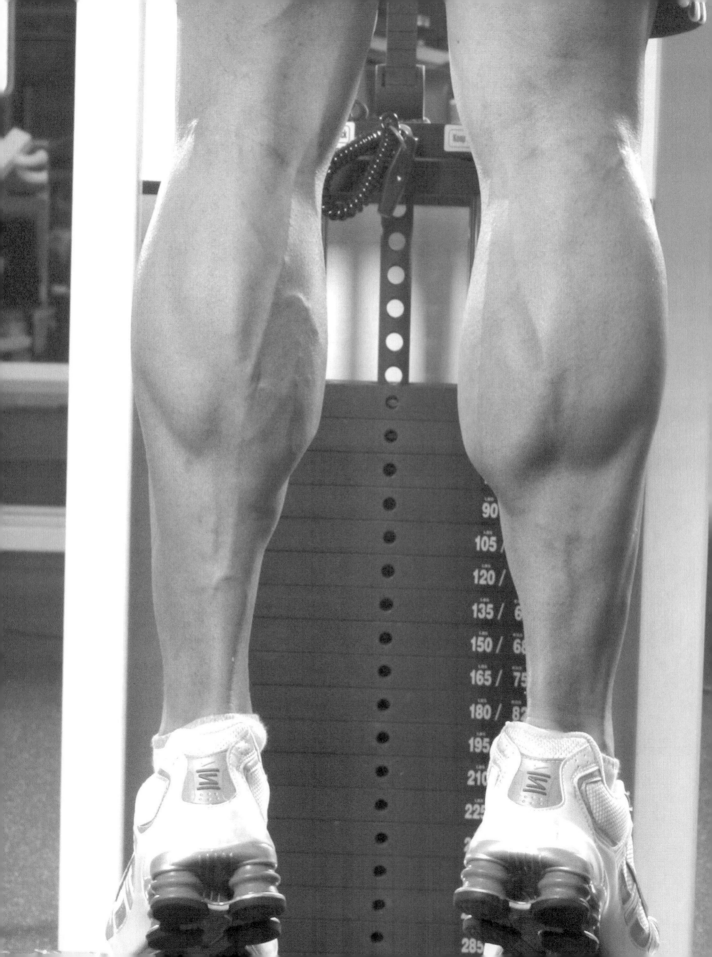

CHAPTER 14

Calf Exercises

Note: *For calves there is really no distinction between basic and isolation exercises*

BASIC EXERCISES

Standing Calf Raises

Calf Press

Donkey Calf Raises

Seated Calf Raises

Tibia Raises

ALTERNATIVE EXERCISES

One-Legged Dumbbell Calf Raises

Two-Legged Dumbbell Calf Raises

Barbell Calf Raises

In this chapter we will cover the execution of all the calf exercises presented in the routines of this program.

The calves are even more neglected than the quadriceps and hamstrings put together. While for the most part, beginning bodybuilders will at least do some leg extensions and curls, they forget to incorporate the very important calf raises.

Diamond-shaped calves are valuable to a complete symmetrical physique. Calves are composed of the gastrocnemius (which makes up most of the calf and over 70% of the lower leg consisting of two heads) and the soleus. The gastrocnemius is located on top of the lower leg, attaching itself above the knee, and the soleus is the muscle underneath, which attaches below the knee. There is also the tibialis anterior which is located on the front of the lower leg by the shinbone. Its main function is to simply lift the heel by flexing the foot. Because of this, calf raises and tibia raises are the way in which the calf muscles are trained.

Foot Stances and Calf Development

There are three foot positions that can be used when performing calf raises:

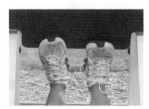 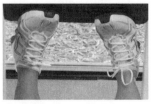 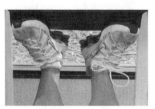

1. Toes straight: Good for overall development.

2. Toes in: Good for maximizing outer head stimulation.

3. Toes out: Good for maximizing inner head stimulation.

Having said this, we will now cover in order of appearance the exercises used on this program and at the end of the chapter I will cover some additional useful exercises that can be used as well in lieu of the ones in the routines above.

Standing Calf Raises

FOOT STANCE: *All stances*

1 Adjust the padded lever of the calf raise machine to fit your height.

2 Place your shoulders under the pads provided and position your toes facing forward (or using any of the two other positions described at the beginning of the chapter). The balls of your feet should be secure on top of the calf block with the heels extending off it. Push the lever up by extending your hips and knees until your torso is standing erect. The knees should be kept with a slight bend; never locked. Toes should be facing forward, outward, or inward as described at the beginning of the chapter. This will be your starting position.

3 Raise your heels as you breathe out by extending your ankles as high as possible and flexing your calves. Ensure that the knee is kept stationary at all times. There should be no bending at any time. Hold the contracted position for a second before you start to go back down.

4 Go back slowly to the starting position as you breathe in by lowering your heels as you bend the ankles until calves are stretched.

5 Repeat for the recommended number of repetitions.

Caution: If you suffer from lower back problems, a better exercise is the calf press because during a standing calf raise the back has to support the weight being lifted. Also, keep your back straight and stationary at all times. Rounding of the back can cause lower back injury.

Variations: There are several other ways to perform a standing calf raise. A barbell or dumbells can be used instead of a machine, one leg or two legs at a time. Refer to the exercise descriptions of these movements below. A Smith machine can be used for calf raises as well.

Notes: Emphasize the stretch portion by pausing a second at the bottom and then continuing the movement. Make sure that you pause a second at the top.

Standing Calf Raises

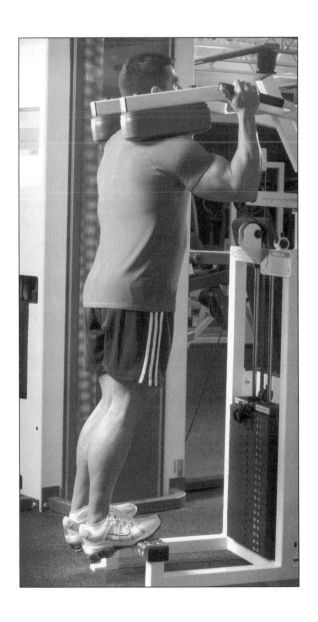

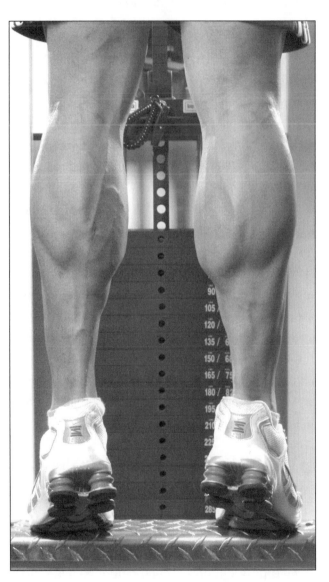

Calf Press

Calf Raises Performed on the Leg Press Machine

FOOT STANCE: *All stances*

1 Using a leg press machine, sit down on the machine and place your legs on the platform directly in front of you at a medium (shoulder width) foot stance.

2 Lower the safety bars holding the weighted platform in place and press the platform all the way up until your legs are fully extended in front of you without locking your knees. (Note: In some leg press units you can leave the safety bars on for increased safety. If your leg press unit allows for this, then this is the preferred method of performing the exercise.) Your torso and the legs should make a perfect 90-degree angle. Now carefully place your toes and balls of your feet on the lower portion of the platform with the heels extending off. Toes should be facing forward, outward, or inward as described at the beginning of the chapter. This will be your starting position.

3 Press on the platform by raising your heels as you breathe out by extending your ankles as high as possible and flexing your calves. Be sure that the knee is kept stationary at all times. There should be no bending at any time. Hold the contracted position for a second before you start to go back down.

4 Go back slowly to the starting position as you breathe in by lowering your heels as you bend the ankles until calves are stretched.

5 Repeat for the recommended number of repetitions.

Caution: Be very cautious as you place the feet in the bottom part of the platform. If you slip and the safety bars are not locked, you could suffer a serious accident.

Variations: You can perform this exercise one leg at a time.

Calf Press

Calf Raises Performed on the Leg Press Machine

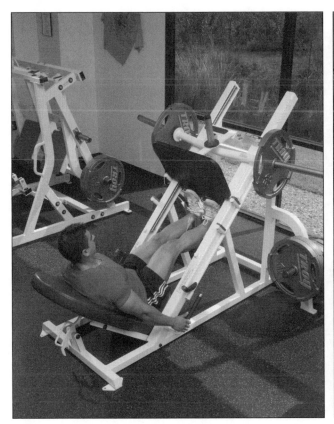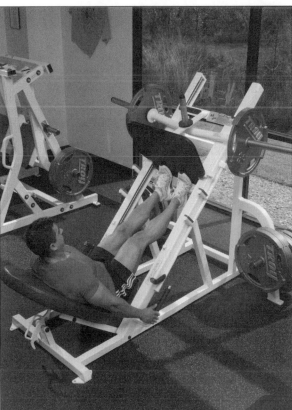

Donkey Calf Raises

FOOT STANCE: *All stances*

❶ For this exercise you will either need access to a donkey calf raise machine or a calf block and a sturdy low bar, as pictured.

❷ After adjusting your weight belt, step up on the calf block with your heels extending off. Align the toes forward, inward, or outward, depending on the area you wish to target, and straighten the knees without locking them. Lean forward and grasp the bar with both hands. This will be your starting position.

❸ Raise your heels as you breathe out by extending your ankles as high as possible and flexing your calves. Be sure that the knees are kept stationary at all times. There should be no bending at any time. Hold the contracted position a second before you start to go back down.

❹ Go back slowly to the starting position as you breathe in by lowering your heels as you bend the ankles until calves are stretched.

❺ Repeat for the recommended number of repetitions.

Donkey Calf Raises

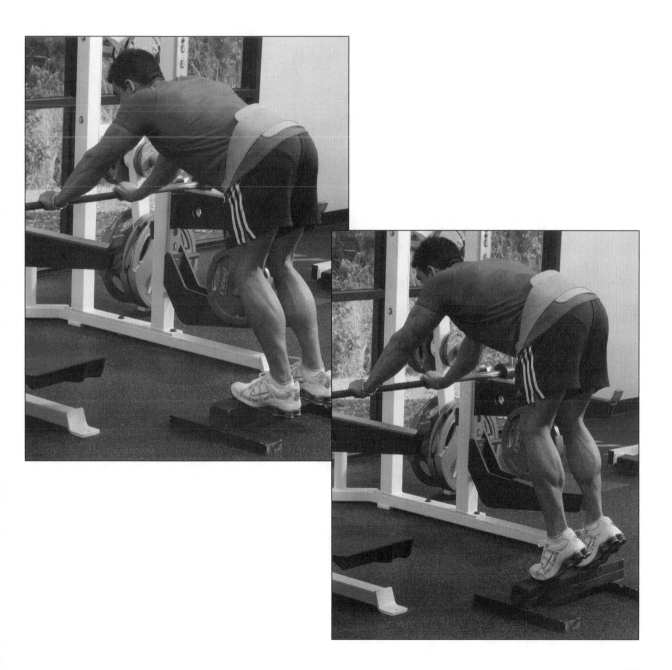

Seated Calf Raises

FOOT STANCE: *All stances*

❶ Sit on the Seated Calf Raise machine and place your toes on the lower portion of the platform with the heels extending off. Choose the toe positioning of your choice (forward, in, or out) as at the beginning of this chapter.

❷ Place your lower thighs under the lever pad, which will need to be adjusted according to the height of your thighs. Now place your hands on top of the lever pad in order to prevent it from slipping forward.

❸ Lift the lever slightly by pushing your heels up and release the safety bar. This will be your starting position.

❹ Slowly lower your heels by bending at the ankles until the calves are fully stretched. Inhale as you perform this movement.

❺ Raise the heels by extending the ankles as high as possible as you contract the calves and breathe out. Hold the top contraction for a second.

❻ Repeat for the recommended number of repetitions.

Seated Calf Raises

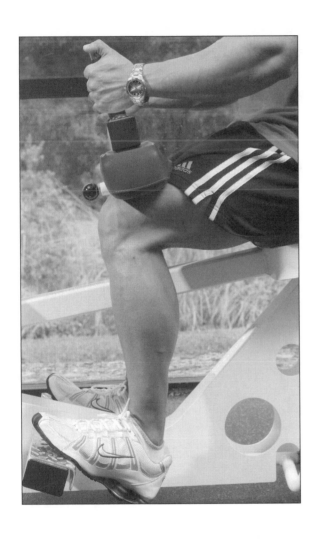
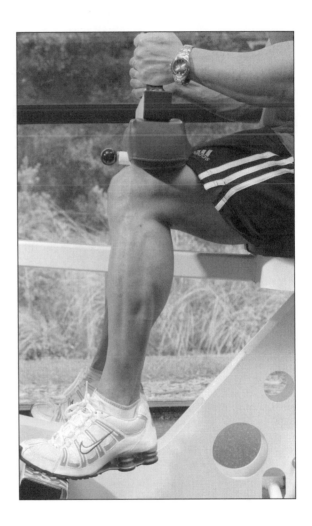

Tibia Raises

① Position your heels on the forward edge of either a calf block or a raised platform. The feet should be placed facing straight ahead, with toes pointing down and legs slightly less than shoulder width apart. Use a fixed object to keep your torso in balance. This will be your starting position.

② Raise the toes towards you as high as you can as you exhale. Hold one second on the contracted position.

③ Lower your toes back to their original position as you inhale.

④ Repeat for the recommended number of times.

Variations: As you get stronger you can hold a dumbbell in between your feet for added resistance.

Tibia Raises

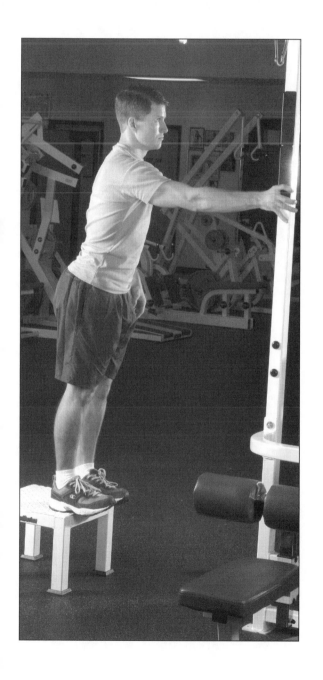

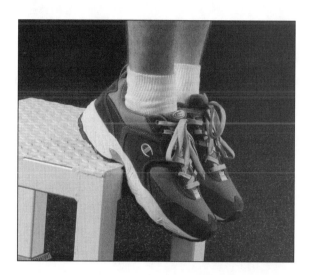

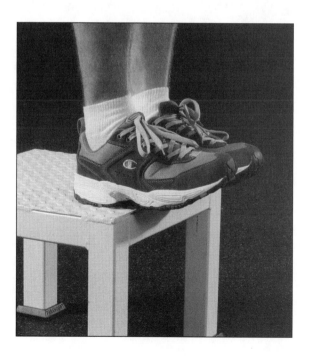

One-Legged Dumbbell Calf Raises

❶ Grasp a dumbbell with your left hand and position the ball of your right foot on a calf block or a raised platform with the heels extending off. The toes should be facing forward.

❷ To keep your body balanced, place your right hand on a fixed object such as a beam on a squat rack. Bend your left knee and lift the leg off the platform.

❸ While exhaling, raise the heel of your right leg by pulling the ankles as high as possible as you contract the calves.

❹ Inhale and lower the heel by returning the ankle to its lowered position.

❺ When you are finished with the right leg, switch the dumbbell to the right hand and perform the exercise with the left leg.

One-Legged Dumbbell Calf Raises

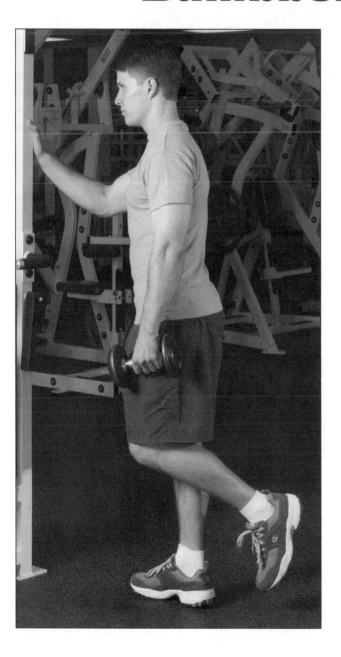
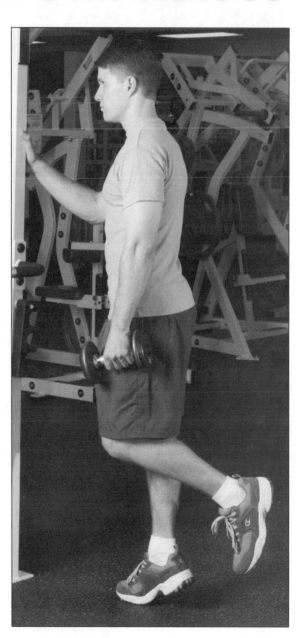

Two-Legged Dumbbell Calf Raises

❶ Stand upright with two dumbbells in your hands by your sides.

❷ Choose the toe position of your preference and raise the heels off the floor as you exhale by contracting the calves. Hold the top contraction for a second.

❸ As you inhale, go back to the starting position by slowly lowering the heels.

❹ Repeat for the recommended number of times.

Note: For this exercise, you won't be able to stretch fully because you are not using a calf block. However, the exercise is still effective. As you become stronger you may need to use wrist wraps to avoid having the dumbbells slip from your hands.

Two-Legged Dumbbell Calf Raises

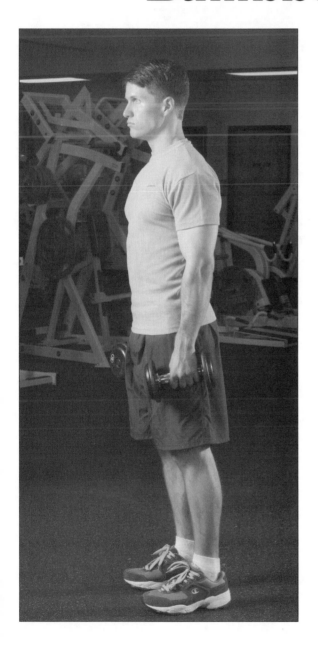 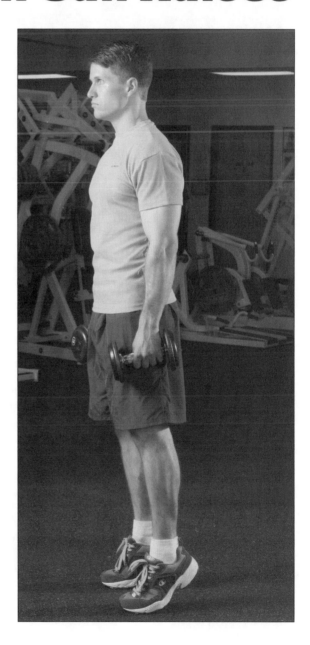

Barbell Calf Raises

❶ Set a barbell on a power rack at the height of your upper chest and secure a calf block properly beneath it.

❷ Place the back of your shoulders under the barbell with both hands to the sides for stability. The balls of your feet should be positioned on the calf block with the heels extending off. Pick the footing preference of your choice.

❸ Lean the barbell against the rack and raise it from the supports by extending the knees and hips. Do not lock your knees and keep your back straight without slouching forward. Support the barbell against the front vertical beams of the squat rack with both hands to your sides. For added safety, you can adjust the side safety pins of the squat rack to the top position just right under the bar.

❹ Exhale and raise your heels by extending your ankles as high as possible and flexing your calves. Your knees should be stationary at all times. Hold the contracted position for a second before you start to go back down.

❺ Inhale and return slowly to the starting position, lowering your heels as you bend the ankles until calves are fully stretched.

Caution: For those with lower back problems, a better exercise is the calf press. Keep your back straight and stationary at all times—rounding of the back can cause lower back injury.

Variations: If no calf block is available you can also perform the exercise without it, but you will be missing the added stretch that the calf block provides.

Barbell Calf Raises

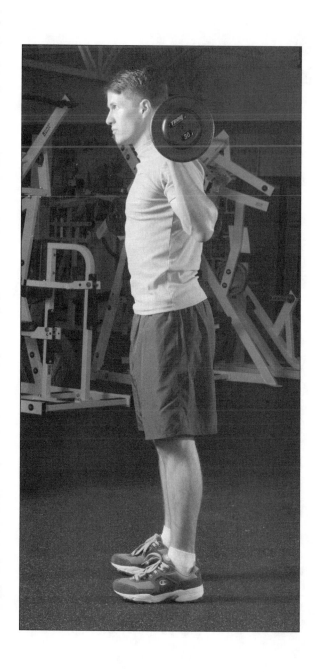 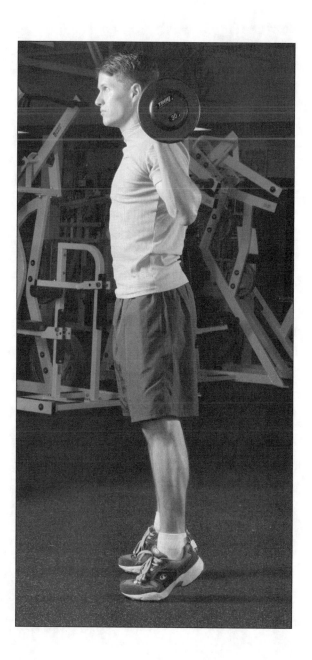

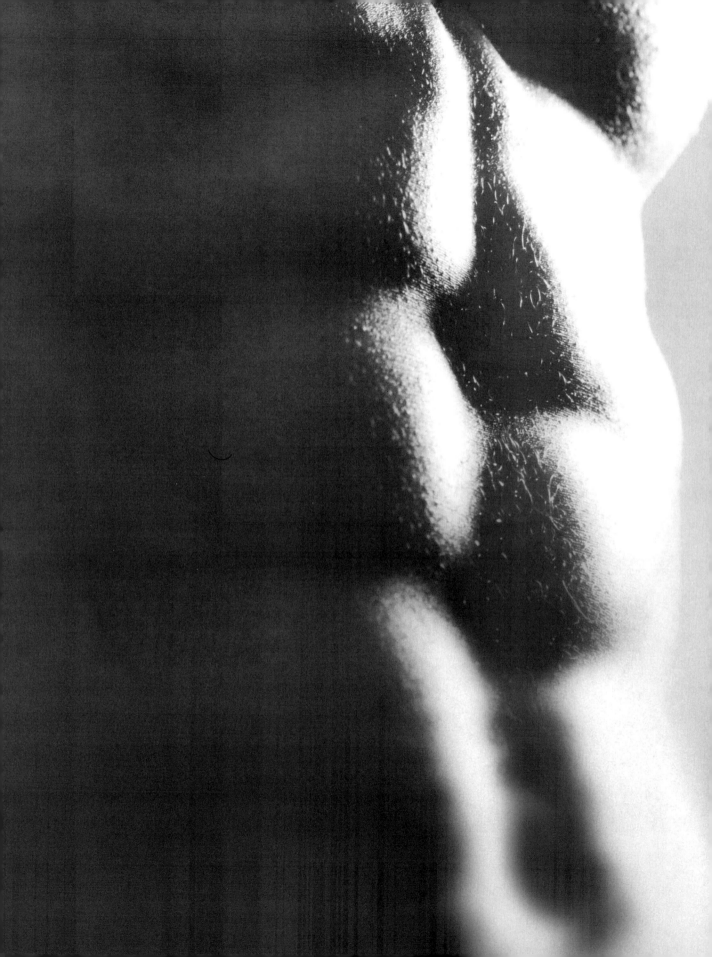

CHAPTER 15
Abdominal Exercises

Note: *For abdominals there is really no distinction between basic and isolation exercises.*

BASIC EXERCISES

Crunches
Lying Leg Raises
Hanging Leg Raises
Bicycle Crunches

ALTERNATIVE EXERCISES

Knee-Ins
V-Ups
Incline Board Partial Sit-Ups
Ab Bench Crunches

In this chapter we will cover the execution of all the abdominal exercises presented in the routines of this program.

While the abdominals are one of the most admired and wanted body parts, most bodybuilders pay no attention whatsoever to them during a mass building phase. This is true even of competitive national athletes. There are three reasons why this is a big mistake:

• The abdominals make up half of your torso so as a result, poor development will lead to lower back pains as the lower back will have to compensate for the strength imbalances created. Think of a tree trunk with a rectangular cut on the front. In such a case, the tree trunk will tend to fall forward. The same thing happens to a body with no abdominal development; it has an unstable trunk.

• Well-developed abdominals increase your strength in exercises like deadlifts, squats and overhead presses. By not training the abdominals you are missing out on growth that could be achieved by higher strength levels on these exercises.

• Finally, by not training the abdominals you are missing out on developing the most visually impressive set of muscles there is. Have you noticed how many commercials these days show guys and gals with a nice set of abs? Food for thought.

The abdominal muscles are arranged in layers stacked on top of each other. The transverse abdominis, or TVA, is the deepest layer; it helps to support the lower back. On top of the TVA, we find the external and internal obliques, which are located on the sides of the torso and whose function is to increase the intra-abdominal pressure necessary for the support of the vertebral column in some exercises such as the squat. In addition, they are the muscle responsible for torso rotation and leaning. Finally comes the muscle that most people refer to as the "six-pack" which is called—the rectus abdominis. The rectus abdominis, is the primary abdominal muscle, which is located at the front of the torso, extending from the sternum down to the top of the pelvis. Its function is to move the torso towards the pelvis/hips.

While during a mass phase the TVA and obliques are stimulated indirectly through the use of basic exercises, the rectus abdominis needs direct stimulation. In order to correctly stimulate this muscle its function needs to be understood.

As we have already mentioned, the function is to pull the upper torso towards the hips when the body is only slightly flexed at the waist. This is the reason why if you are doing a sit-up, any additional torso movement done past the initial 30 degrees from the floor will not stimulate the abs; instead the hips will be the ones that will complete the movement. Because of this, partial sit-ups performed with the torso moving up to 30 degrees and crunches are great allies in our quest to achieve great abs.

However, if you really want to maximally stimulate the abdominals and prevent lower back problems, you need to also consider that the anatomy of the rectus abdominis. If you do not bend your torso backwards by around 15 to 20 degrees then you won't be able to get a full abdominal stretch. As a result, this will prevent you from achieving full development and strength benefits. Since the floor only provides a flat surface, your abs will not get maximal stimulation. They will also not learn how to properly contract and protect your back when your body is bent backwards (for example when advanced bodybuilders perform exercises like standing military presses).

The only way to get around this is by using a swiss ball (also known as exercise ball or medicine ball). A swiss ball will allow you to get the necessary backward bend that your torso needs in order to maximally stimulate your abs. Because of this, crunches performed on an exercise ball are the way in which I recommend you perform this exercise.

Since the rectus abdominis also has muscles in the lower region that help maintain proper postural alignment, it becomes necessary to include leg raises performed on the swiss ball (make sure that you hold to a stationary sturdy object) as this exercise will allow you to go below the neutral (flat) position. Another good lower abdominal exercise is the hanging leg raise. The key for maximal stimulation in this exercise is to roll the pelvis slightly backwards at the beginning of the movement.

One last thing that I want to cover before presenting the exercise descriptions is the subject of repetitions. While it has been long believed that high repetitions are the key to strengthening abs this is a misconception. Much to our surprise, studies indicate that the rectus abdominis is composed mainly of fast-twitch fibers. These fibers (as opposed to the slow twitch, endurance fibers), are composed of the strongest types of muscle fibers and are thus designed for short bouts of explosive hard work. Because of this, fast-twitch fibers respond best to heavy weight/low repetition work. Therefore, performing more than 15 repetitions per set on your abdominal exercises will be largely a waste of time! Abdominal definition is more a function of body fat percentage, something that through dietary manipulations and some cardiovascular activity can be reduced. Only when the body fat is below 10% can we start seeing the abdominals, with awesome definition displayed at 6%. Then again, for hardgainers, typically abdominal definition is usually not an issue as their body fat is kept low year round.

Regarding training frequency, we need to keep in mind that fast twitch fibers take longer to recover. Therefore, we need to train these muscles as we train any other muscles and give them the rest they need. Interesting things science can teach us!

Crunches

1 Sit on an exercise ball with your lower back curvature pressed against the surface of the ball. Your feet should be bent at the knee and pressed firmly against the floor. The upper torso should be hanging off the top of the ball. The arms should either be kept alongside the body or crossed on top of your chest as these positions avoid neck strain (as opposed to the hands behind the back of the head position).

2 Lower your torso into a stretch position, keeping the neck stationary at all times. This will be your starting position.

3 With the hips stationary, flex the waist by contracting the abdominals and curl the shoulders and trunk upward until you feel a nice contraction on your abdominals. The arms should simply slide up the side of your legs if you have them at the side, or just stay on top of your chest if you have them crossed. The lower back should always stay in contact with the ball. Exhale as you perform this movement and hold the contraction for a second.

4 As you inhale, go back to the starting position.

5 Repeat for the recommended number of repetitions.

Caution: Perform this exercise slowly and deliberately as it takes some getting used to. Also, do not be hasty and try to use weights the first time; you'll have enough on your hands learning how to balance yourself. Also, if balance is an issue I recommend having a spotter next to you and also placing each of your feet under a 100-lb dumbbell for added stability. As you get more advanced you can hold a dumbbell or a weight on top of your chest. However, you have to be very careful when adding weight to this exercise; if you add too much too quickly you could get a hernia.

Variations: You can perform this exercise with a low pulley behind you with a rope attached to its end. In this manner you can more easily add resistance easier. For this variation, you will need to hold on to the the rope throughout the movement. I like to bring my arms forward to the point where the upper arms are almost parallel to my torso and the lower arms are facing back holding the rope.

Notes: On the crunches, emphasize the stretch at the bottom and pause for a second while contracting at the top. If you choose to add weight, you can add resistance by using a cable pulley with a rope at the end from behind you, or holding a plate with your arms extended in front of you.

Crunches

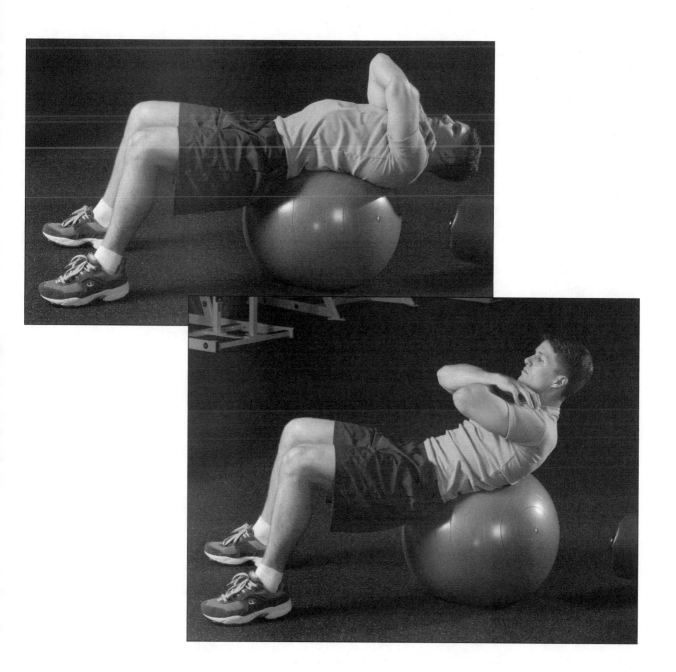

Lying Leg Raises

1 Sit on an exercise ball with your lower back curvature pressed against the surface of the ball. Hold on to a fixed and sturdy object behind you such as one of the beams from a squat rack. Your feet should be straight in front of you. The upper torso should be hanging off the top of the ball with the arms behind you holding on to the fixed object.

2 Raises your legs to where they are off the floor but slightly below parallel to ensure a full stretch of the abdominal region. The pelvis should be rolled slightly backwards. This will be your starting position.

3 Raise your legs until the torso makes a 90-degree angle with the legs. Exhale as you perform this movement and hold the contraction for a second or so.

4 Go back slowly to the starting position as you breathe in.

5 Repeat for the recommended number of repetitions.

Caution: Perform this exercise slowly and deliberately as it takes some getting used to. Also, do not be hasty and try to use weights the first time; you'll have enough on your hands learning how to balance yourself. As you get more advanced you can hold a dumbbell in between your feet or attach a pulley to them for added resistance. However, you have to be very careful when adding weight to this exercise; if you add too much too quickly you could get a hernia.

Notes: You must be very careful when adding weight to this exercise, because too much added too quickly could result in a hernia.

While exercising with the lying leg raises, pause at the top of the contraction for a second, then lower slowly.

Lying Leg Raises

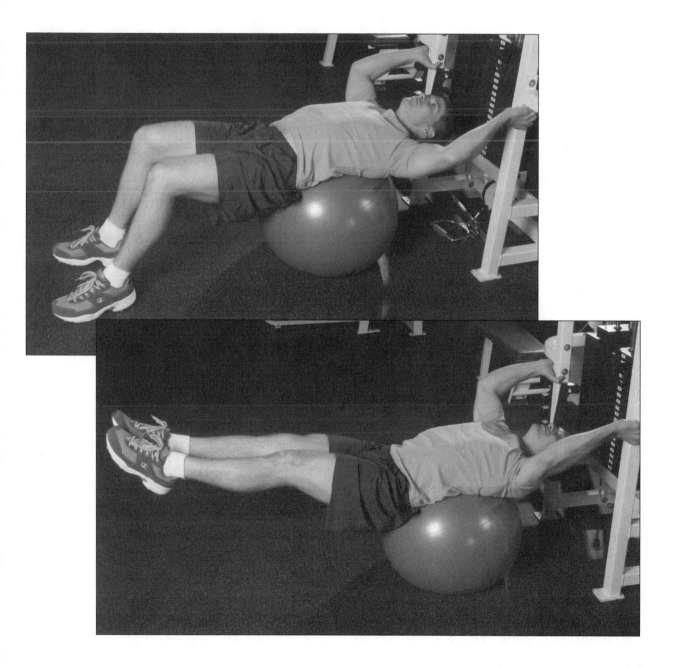

Hanging Leg Raises

1 Hang with both arms fully extended using either a wide or a medium grip. The legs should be straight down with the pelvis rolled slightly backward. This will be your starting position.

2 Raise your legs until the torso makes a 90-degree angle with the legs. Exhale as you perform this movement and hold the contraction for a second or so.

3 Go back slowly to the starting position as you breathe in.

4 Repeat for the recommended number of repetitions.

Caution: Perform this exercise slowly and deliberately as it takes some getting used to. Also, do not be hasty and try to use weights on the first time; you'll have enough on your hands holding your weight and also learning how to balance yourself so that you avoid swinging your torso. As you get more advanced you can hold a dumbbell in between your feet. However, you have to be very careful when adding weight to this exercise; if you add too much too quickly you could get a hernia.

Variation: This exercise can also be performed using a vertical bench that makes the exercise easier by supporting your upper back in place and by allowing you to hold yourself by placing your elbows and arms on the side pads.

Hanging Leg Raises

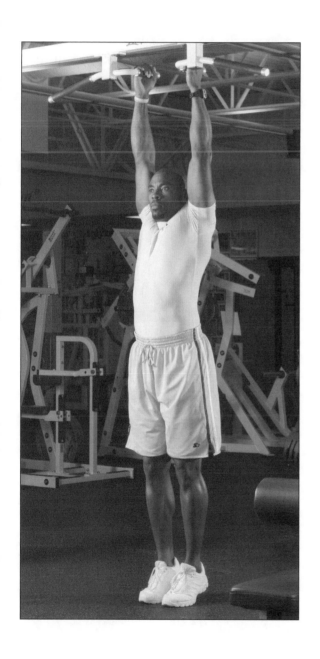
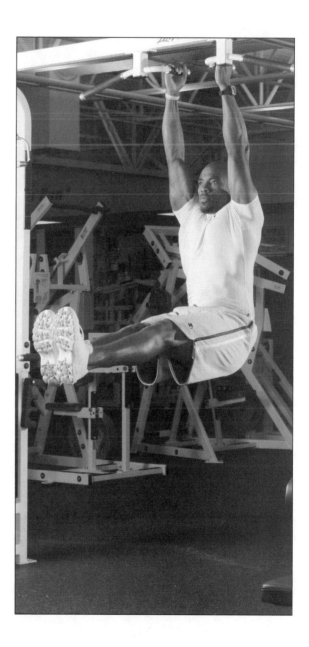

Bicycle Crunches

❶ Lie flat on the floor with your lower back pressed to the ground. For this exercise, you will need to put your hands behind your head. Be careful not to strain with the neck as you perform it. Now lift your shoulders into the crunch position.

❷ Bring knees up to where they are perpendicular to the floor, with your lower legs parallel to the floor. This will be your starting position.

❸ Now simultaneously, slowly go through a cycle pedal motion, kicking forward with the right leg and bringing in the knee of the left leg. Bring your right elbow close to your left knee by crunching to the side as you breathe out.

❹ Go back to the initial position as you breathe in.

❺ Crunch to the opposite side as you cycle your legs and bring your left elbow closer to your right knee and exhale.

❻ Continue alternating in this manner until all of the recommended repetitions for each side have been completed.

Notes: While you cannot add resistance to this exercise you can concentrate on perfect execution and slow speed.

Bicycle Crunches

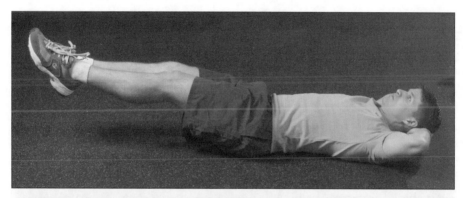

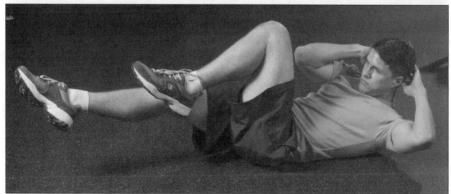

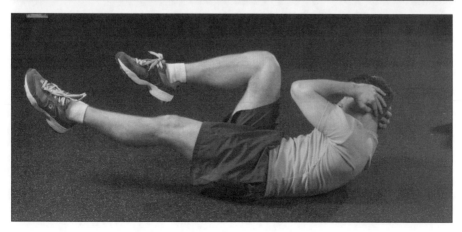

Knee-Ins

1 Sit on a bench with your legs stretched out in front of you with your knees slightly bent and your arms holding on to the sides of the bench. You should be leaning backwards at a 45-degree angle from the bench.

2 Exhale while bringing your knees in toward you, simultaneously moving your torso closer to them. Your ankles should end near the bench.

3 Pause at the top, and return to the starting position, inhaling as you do so.

Variations: To make this easier, try it on a mat on the floor with your arms out to the sides. To make this more difficult, hold a dumbbell between your feet or attach a pulley to them for added resistance. You must, however, be very careful when adding weight to this exercise to avoid injury.

Knee-Ins

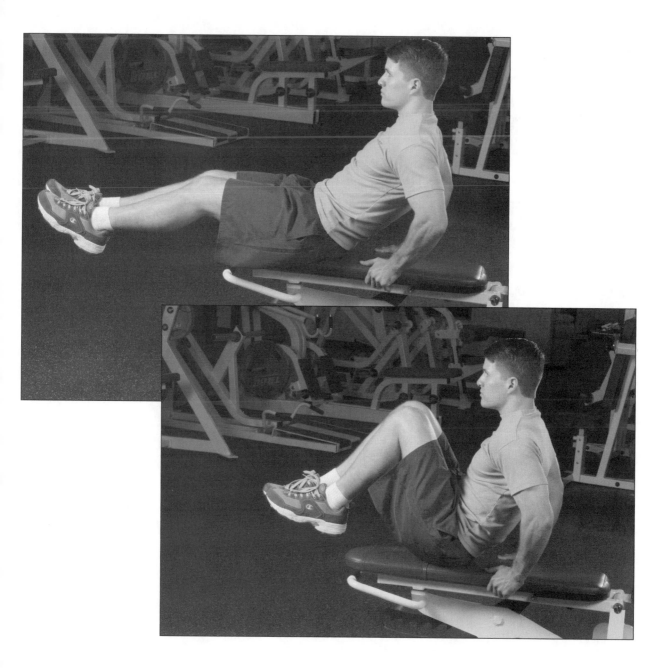

V-Ups

1 Sit on a bench with your legs stretched out in front of you with your knees slightly bent and your arms holding on to the sides of the bench. You should be leaning backwards at a 45-degree angle from the bench.

2 Exhale while bringing your legs in toward you, simultaneously moving your torso closer to your knees. Your ankles should end high above your head.

3 Pause at the top and return to the starting position, inhaling as you do.

Variations: To make this easier, try it on a mat on the floor with your arms to the sides. To make this more advanced, hold a dumbbell between your feet or attach a pulley to them for added resistance. You must, however, be very careful when adding weight to this exercise to avoid injury. You can also perform the exercise by lifting the arms and the torso off the floor as you also raise your legs. This is one of the most challenging abdominal exercises and can be stressful on the lower back.

V-Ups

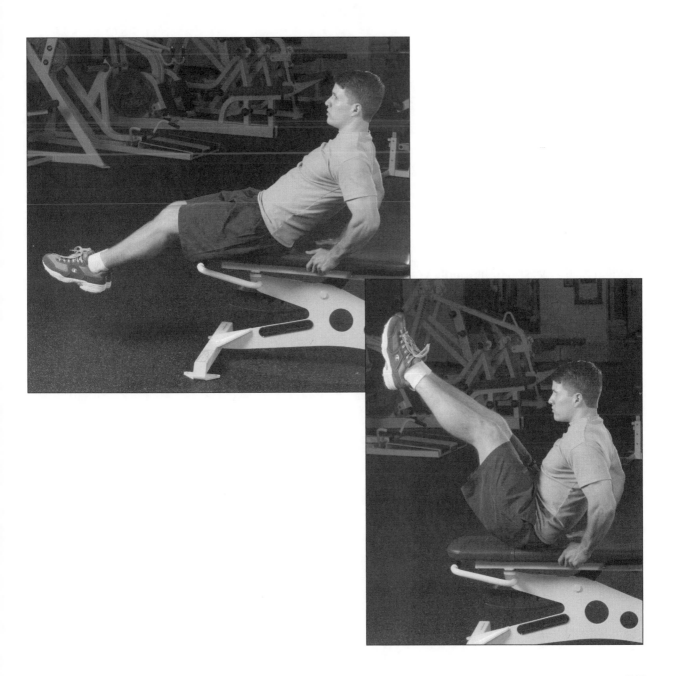

Incline Board Partial Sit-Ups

❶ Set the abdominal board to an incline. The more advanced you are, the steeper the incline you should choose. Hook your feet under the foot brace provided and lie on it with your hands crossed on top of your chest or kept alongside the body.

❷ As you exhale, raise your torso from bench by bending at the waist and hips until you achieve a 30-degree angle between the torso and the bench.

❸ Slowly return to the starting position as you inhale.

Caution: This may be hard on the lower back, so avoid it if you have an unhealthy back. Avoid performing this exercise by swinging your torso as this leads to injury.

Variations: Varying the angle of this exercise by choosing smaller or steeper inclines can increase or decrease the difficulty. Beginners should always start with no angle. As you become more advanced, weight can be added by holding a plate to your chest.

Incline Board Partial Sit-Ups

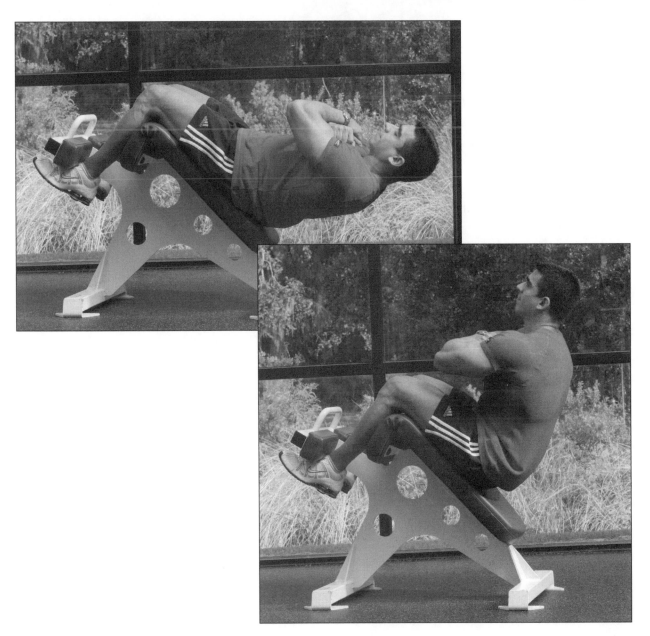

Ab Bench Crunches

❶ For this exercise you will need a bench created by Ironman called the Ab Bench. This bench has a rounded back that allows for full stretch of the abdominals. To use it, sit with your back on the rounded pad and hold onto the handlebars. Your feet should be firm on the ground and torso should be tilted back to stretch the abdominals.

❷ As you exhale, pull your torso forward and maintain full contact with the back pad. Hold the contraction for a second.

❸ While inhaling, slowly return to the starting position.

Caution: As always, be very careful when adding weight to this exercise; if you add too much too quickly you could injure yourself.

Ab Bench Crunches

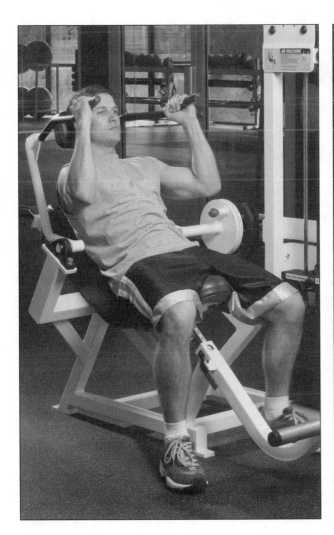
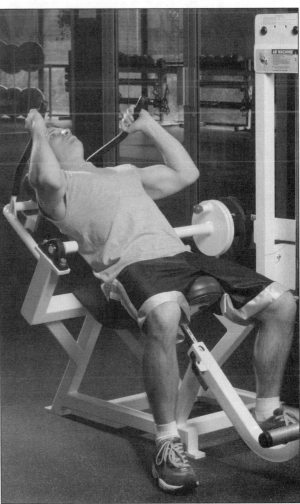

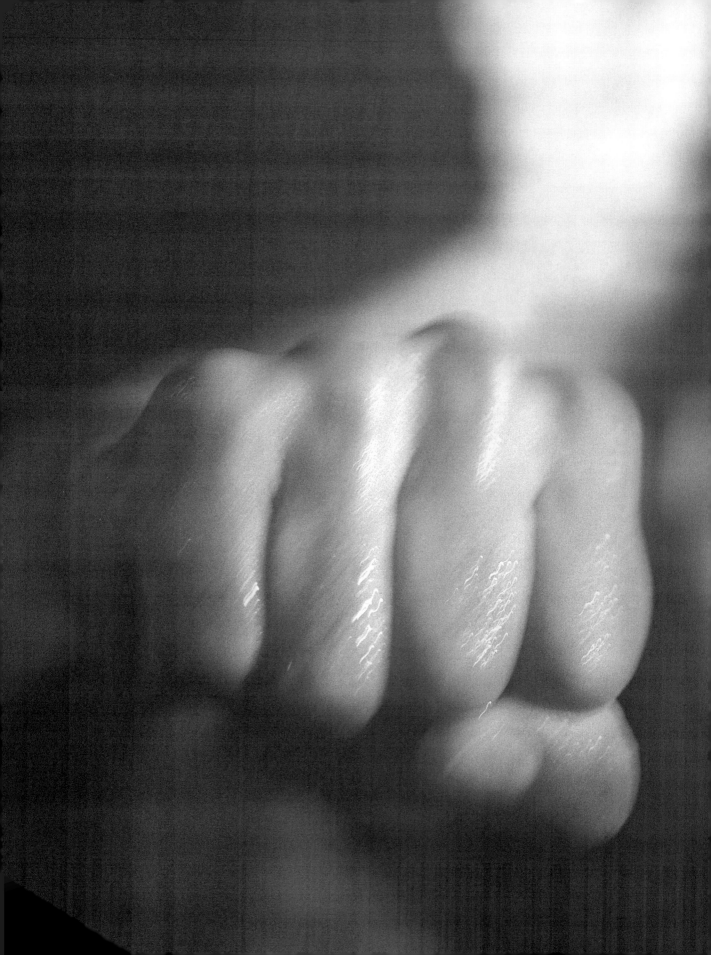

CONCLUSION

Conclusion

In order to go on a trip and reach the destination, you need to know where you are at and where you are heading to. In this book I have provided a road map to get you from your current point of development to the point that you desire. The topics of training, nutrition, supplementation and recuperation should not longer be an unknown and confusing science, as now you are armed with the information that you need to do things correctly. It is now time to use your determination and apply this new knowledge that you have gained in order to achieve your goals. Remember that knowledge without action is only wasted knowledge. Only applied knowledge is power. So stop reading, go to the gym and apply what you have learned. Soon you will look at the mirror and not recognize the person staring back at you.

Wishing you the best in your fitness endeavors!

Best of Health,
Hugo A. Rivera
President
HR Fitness Inc.
http://www.hrfit.net

APPENDIX A: MEAL PLAN SCHEDULE AND FOOD GROUP TABLES

Use the caloric matrix to find your daily nutrient requirements by identifying your body weight.

Meal Plan Schedule

Divide the total values obtained by six to create a diet using the food group tables. Plug the values obtained in the corresponding spaces below. Your meal plan will consist of breakfast, lunch, and dinner, with three snacks in between. The snacks can be in the form of real food or protein shakes (your choice).

Notes: The schedule is based on an 8 a.m.–5 p.m. job but you can modify it to suit your individual needs. If you work out at any other time than the evening, simply move the

BODY WEIGHT	CALORIES	PROTEINS	FATS	CARBOHYDRATES
100	2400	150	67	300
110	2640	165	73	330
120	2880	180	80	360
130	3120	195	87	390
140	3360	210	93	420
150	3600	225	100	450
160	3840	240	107	480
170	4080	255	113	510
180	4320	270	120	540
190	4560	285	127	570
200	4800	300	133	600
210	5040	315	140	630
220	5280	330	147	660
230	5520	345	153	690
240	5760	360	160	720
250	6000	375	167	750
260	6240	390	173	780
270	6480	405	180	810
280	6720	420	187	840
290	6960	435	193	870
300	7200	450	200	900

post workout meal to the time at which you are done working out and continue with the next meal following. For instance, if you work out at 10 a.m., then your post workout meal will be at 11 or 11:30 a.m. (at the latest) and then the following meal will be your lunch 2 to 3 hours later. The mid-morning snack then will become your late evening snack to be consumed around 9 p.m.

FOOD GROUP TABLES

MEAL 1 *(7:00 a.m.)* **BREAKFAST**
Choose _____ grams from Group A
Choose _____ grams from Group B
Choose _____ grams from Group E

MEAL 2 *(10:00 a.m.)* **MID-MORNING**
Choose _____ grams from Group A
Choose _____ grams from Group C
Choose _____ grams from Group E

MEAL 3 *(12:30 p.m.)* **LUNCH**
Choose _____ grams from Group A
Choose _____ grams from Group B
Choose _____ grams from Group D
Choose _____ grams from Group E

MEAL 4 *(3:00 p.m.)* **MID-AFTERNOON**
Choose _____ grams from Group A
Choose _____ grams from Group C
Choose _____ grams from Group E

MEAL 5 *(5:30 p.m.)* **EARLY DINNER**
Choose _____ grams from Group A
Choose _____ grams from Group B
Choose _____ grams from Group D
Choose _____ grams from Group E

WORKOUT: 7:30 p.m.—8:30 p.m.

MEAL 5 *(9:00 p.m.)* **POST WORKOUT MEAL**
Choose _____ grams from Group A
Choose _____ grams from Group C

GROUP A - PROTEIN

FOOD	GRAMS	FOOD	GRAMS
Chicken breast (3.5 oz broiled)	33	Whitefish (3.5 oz broiled)	31
Tuna (packed in water, 3.5 oz)	35	Halibut (3.5 oz broiled)	31
Turkey breast (3.5 oz broiled)	28	Cod (3.5 oz broiled)	31
Whey protein powder (2 scoops)	22	Round steak (3.5 oz broiled)	33
10 egg whites	35	Top sirloin (4 oz)	35

Note: These weights are for uncooked portions

GROUP B - CARBOHYDRATE (COMPLEX, STARCHY)

FOOD	GRAMS	FOOD	GRAMS
Baked potato (3.5 oz broiled)	21	Lentils (1 cup dry, cooked)	38
Plain oatmeal (1/2 cup dry)	27	Grits (1/4 cup dry)	31
Whole wheat bread	13	Chickpeas (1 cup cooked)	45
(limit if trying to go below 10% body fat		Brown rice (2/3 cup cooked)	30
as wheat contains pythoestrogens)		Cream of Rice (1/4 cup dry, post workout only)	38
Pita bread (1 piece)	33	Sweet potato (4 oz)	28

GROUP C - CARBOHYDRATE (SIMPLE)

FOOD	GRAMS	FOOD	GRAMS
Apple (1)	15	Banana (6 oz, post workout only)	27
Cantaloupe (1/2)	25	Grapes (1 cup, post workout only)	14
Strawberries (1 cup)	9	Grapefruit (1/2)	12
Orange (1)	15	Tangerine (1)	9
Pear (1)	27	Cherries (1 cup)	22
Lemon (1)	5	Nectarine (1)	16
Peach (1)	10	Skim milk (1 cup, preferably post workout only)	13

GROUP D - CARBOHYDRATE (COMPLEX, FIBROUS)

FOOD (10 oz serving)	GRAMS	FOOD (10 oz serving)	GRAMS
Asparagus	5	Yellow squash	12
Broccoli	17	Green beans	23
Cabbage	6	Cauliflower	12
Celery	6	Cucumber	7
Mushrooms	6	Lettuce	7
Red or Green peppers	15	Tomato	5
Spinach	3	Zucchini	13

GROUP E - CARBOHYDRATE (COMPLEX, FIBROUS)

MONOUNSATURATED (1 TABLESPOON)	GRAMS	POLYUNSATURATED (1 TABLESPOON)	GRAMS
Extra Virgin Olive Oil	14	Flaxseed Oil	14
Natural Peanut Butter	8	Fish Oils	14

Sample Meal Plan for a 100-Pound Hardgainer

Since a 100-lb athlete requires 2400 calories, 150 grams of protein, 67 grams of fats and 300 grams of carbohydrates, the meal plan requirements will look like the following:

Notes:

• Notice that since fats came out to a value of 13.4 grams per meal, I just rounded up to 14 grams.

• Since there are incidental nutrients like a few extra grams of protein in the carb sources etc, the caloric value will be higher than 2400.

• Remember that fibrous carbs, group D, do not factor into our carbohydrate calculations. The way to figure out this nutrient is just to add anywhere between 10 and 15 grams of them at lunch and at dinner time.

• Finally, note that the serving sizes do not exactly contain the macronutrient gram amounts recommended for each meal as there is a +/- 5 gram variation. These small variations will not affect your results in any way as for most instances I erred on the side of more grams than less.

BREAKFAST (7:00 A.M.)

CHOOSE   25   GRAMS FROM GROUP A
CHOOSE   50   GRAMS FROM GROUP B
CHOOSE   14   GRAMS FROM GROUP E

Group A: 7 egg whites (can be from Egg Beaters or any other brand) or 25 grams from whey protein

Group B: 1 cup of oatmeal or 3/8 of a cup of grits or 6 tablespoons of Cream of Wheat (farina)

Group E: 1 tablespoon of extra virgin canned olive oil

MID-MORNING SNACK (10:00 A.M.)

CHOOSE   25   GRAMS FROM GROUP A
CHOOSE   50   GRAMS FROM GROUP C
CHOOSE   14   GRAMS FROM GROUP E

Group A: 1 scoop of whey protein powder (if 1 scoop approximates 25 grams) or 3 oz of chicken or turkey

Group C: 1 cantaloupe or 16 oz of skim milk if doing a protein shake (note that this amount has 18 grams of protein and 26 grams of simple carbs already so you need to adjust your serving size of powder and fruit) with 1 cantaloupe

Group E: 2 tablespoons of natural peanut butter

LUNCH (12:30 P.M.)

CHOOSE   25   GRAMS FROM GROUP A
CHOOSE   50   GRAMS FROM GROUP B
CHOOSE   15   GRAMS FROM GROUP D
CHOOSE   14   GRAMS FROM GROUP E

Group A: 3 oz of salmon

Group B: 1-1/4 cup of cooked rice

Group D: 1 can of low-sodium green beans

Group E: The salmon already has the fish oils in it so no need to add extra oils

MID-AFTERNOON (3:00 P.M.)

CHOOSE   25   GRAMS FROM GROUP A
CHOOSE   50   GRAMS FROM GROUP C
CHOOSE   14   GRAMS FROM GROUP E

Group A: 1 scoop of whey protein powder (if 1 scoop approximates 25 grams) or 3 oz of chicken or turkey

Group C: 1 cantaloupe or 16 oz of skim milk if doing a protein shake (note that this amount has 18 grams of protein and 26 grams of simple carbs already so you would need to adjust your serving size of powder and fruit) with 1 cantaloupe

Group E: 1 tablespoon of Flax Oil (could be mixed on the drink)

EARLY DINNER (5:30 P.M.)

CHOOSE   25   GRAMS FROM GROUP A
CHOOSE   50   GRAMS FROM GROUP B
CHOOSE   15   GRAMS FROM GROUP D
CHOOSE   14   GRAMS FROM GROUP E

Group A: 3 oz of top sirloin round steak

Group B: 1-1/4 cup of cooked pasta (semolina)

Group D: 10 oz of fresh broccoli

Group E: The steak has some saturated fats so no need to add fats to this meal.

WORKOUT: 7:30 P.M.–8:30 P.M.

POST WORKOUT MEAL-PROTEIN RECOVERY DRINK (9:00 P.M.)

CHOOSE   25   GRAMS FROM GROUP A
CHOOSE   50   GRAMS FROM GROUP C

Group A: Whey protein (preferably isolate)

Group C: 4 cups of grapes or 12 oz of banana

HARDGAINERS

Sample Meal Plan for a 150 Pound Hardgainer

Since a 150-lb athlete requires 3600 calories, 225 grams of protein, 100 grams of fats, and 450 grams of carbohydrates, the meal plan requirements will look like the following:

Notes:
• Since there are incidental nutrients like a few extra grams of protein in the carb sources etc, the caloric value will be higher than 3600.

• Remember that fibrous carbs, group D, does not factor into our carbohydrate calculations. The way to figure out this nutrient is just to add anywhere between 10-15 grams of them at Lunch and at Dinner time.

BREAKFAST (7:00 A.M.)

CHOOSE 38   GRAMS FROM GROUP A
CHOOSE 75   GRAMS FROM GROUP B
CHOOSE 20   GRAMS FROM GROUP E

Group A: 11 egg whites (can be from egg beaters or any other brand) or 38 grams from whey protein

Group B: 1-1/2 cup of oatmeal or 6/8 of a cup of grits or 9 tablespoons of cream of wheat (farina)

Group E: 1-1/3 Tablespoon of Extra Virgin canned Olive Oil

MID-MORNING SNACK (10:00 A.M.)

CHOOSE 38   GRAMS FROM GROUP A
CHOOSE 75   GRAMS FROM GROUP C
CHOOSE 20   GRAMS FROM GROUP E

Group A: 1-1/2 scoops of whey protein powder (if 1 scoop approximates 25 grams) or 4 oz of chicken or turkey

Group C: 1 cantaloupe and 6 oz banana or 16 oz of skim milk if doing a protein shake (note that this amount has 18 grams of protein and 26 grams of simple carbs already so you would need to adjust your serving size of powder and fruit) with 1 cantaloupe and 6 oz banana.

Group E: 2-1/2 tablespoons of natural peanut butter

LUNCH (12:30 P.M.)

CHOOSE 38   GRAMS FROM GROUP A
CHOOSE 75   GRAMS FROM GROUP B
CHOOSE 15   GRAMS FROM GROUP D
CHOOSE 20   GRAMS FROM GROUP E

Group A: 4 oz of salmon

Group B: 2 cups of cooked rice

Group D: 1 can of low sodium green beans

Group E: the salmon already has the fish oils in it so no need to add extra oils

MID-AFTERNOON (3:00 P.M.)

CHOOSE 38   GRAMS FROM GROUP A
CHOOSE 75   GRAMS FROM GROUP C
CHOOSE 20   GRAMS FROM GROUP E

Group A: 1-1/2 scoops of whey protein powder (if 1 scoop approximates 25 grams) or 4 oz of chicken or turkey

Group C: 1 cantaloupe and 6 oz banana or 16 oz of skim milk if doing a protein shake (note that this amount has 18 grams of protein and 26 grams of simple carbs already so you would need to adjust your serving size of powder and fruit) with 1 cantaloupe and 6 oz banana.

Group E: 1-1/2 tablespoon of flax oil (could be mixed in the drink)

EARLY DINNER (5:30 P.M.)

CHOOSE 38   GRAMS FROM GROUP A
CHOOSE 75   GRAMS FROM GROUP B
CHOOSE 15   GRAMS FROM GROUP D
CHOOSE 20   GRAMS FROM GROUP E

Group A: 4 oz of top sirloin round steak

Group B: 1-3/4 cup of cooked pasta (semolina)

Group D: 10 oz of fresh broccoli

Group E: the steak has some saturated fats so no need to add fats to this meal.

WORKOUT: 7:30P.M.–8:30P.M.

POST WORKOUT MEAL-PROTEIN RECOVERY DRINK (9:00 PM)

CHOOSE 38   GRAMS FROM GROUP A
CHOOSE 75   GRAMS FROM GROUP C

Group A: 20 grams of protein from whey protein (preferably isolate)

Group C: 16 oz skim milk (note that this amount has 18 grams of protein and 26 grams of simple carbs already so you would need to adjust your serving size of protein powder) and 12 oz of banana

Sample Meal Plan for a 200 Pound Hardgainer

Since a 150 lb athlete requires 4800 calories, 300 grams of protein, 133 grams of fats, and 600 grams of carbohydrates, the meal plan requirements will look like the following:

Notes:

• Since there are incidental nutrients like a few extra grams of protein in the carb sources etc, the caloric value will be higher than 3600.

• Remember that fibrous carbs, group D, do not factor into our carbohydrate calculations. The way to figure out this nutrient is just to add anywhere between 10–15 grams of them at lunch and at dinner time.

BREAKFAST (7:00 A.M.)

CHOOSE	50	GRAMS FROM GROUP A
CHOOSE	100	GRAMS FROM GROUP B
CHOOSE	27	GRAMS FROM GROUP E

Group A: 14 egg whites (can be from Egg Beaters or any other brand) or 50 grams from whey protein

Group B: 2 cups of oatmeal or 3/4 of a cup of grits or 12 tablespoons of Cream of Wheat (farina)

Group E: 2 tablespoons of extra virgin canned olive oil

MID-MORNING SNACK (10:00 A.M.)

CHOOSE	50	GRAMS FROM GROUP A
CHOOSE	100	GRAMS FROM GROUP C
CHOOSE	27	GRAMS FROM GROUP E

Group A: 2 scoops of whey protein powder (if 1 scoop approximates 25 grams) or 6 oz of chicken or turkey

Group C: 2 cantaloupes or 32 oz of skim milk if doing a protein shake (note that this amount has 36 grams of protein and 52 grams of simple carbs already so you would need to adjust your serving size of powder and fruit) with 1 cantaloupe.

Group E: 4 tablespoons of natural peanut butter

LUNCH (12:30 P.M.)

CHOOSE	50	GRAMS FROM GROUP A
CHOOSE	100	GRAMS FROM GROUP B
CHOOSE	15	GRAMS FROM GROUP D
CHOOSE	27	GRAMS FROM GROUP E

Group A: 6 oz of salmon

Group B: 2-1/2 cup of cooked rice

Group D: 1 can of low sodium green beans

Group E: the salmon already has the fish oils in it so no need to add extra oils.

MID-AFTERNOON (3:00 P.M.)

CHOOSE	50	GRAMS FROM GROUP A
CHOOSE	100	GRAMS FROM GROUP C
CHOOSE	27	GRAMS FROM GROUP E

Group A: 2 scoops of whey protein powder (if 1 scoop approximates 25 grams) or 6 oz of chicken or turkey

Group C: 2 cantaloupes or 32 oz of skim milk if doing a protein shake (note that this amount has 36 grams of protein and 52 grams of simple carbs already so you would need to adjust your serving size of powder and fruit) with only 1 cantaloupe

Group E: 2 Tablespoons of Flax Oil (could be mixed on the drink)

EARLY DINNER (5:30 P.M.)

CHOOSE	50	GRAMS FROM GROUP A
CHOOSE	100	GRAMS FROM GROUP B
CHOOSE	15	GRAMS FROM GROUP D
CHOOSE	27	GRAMS FROM GROUP E

Group A: 6 oz of top sirloin round steak

Group B: 2-1/2 cups of cooked pasta (semolina)

Group D: 10 oz of fresh broccoli

Group E: The steak has some saturated fats so no need to add fats to this meal.

WORKOUT: 7:30P.M.-8:30P.M.

POST WORKOUT MEAL PROTEIN RECOVERY DRINK (9:00 P.M.)

CHOOSE	50	GRAMS FROM GROUP A
CHOOSE	100	GRAMS FROM GROUP C

Group A: whey protein (preferably isolate)

Group C: 32 oz skim milk (note that this amount has 36 grams of protein and 52 grams of simple carbs already so you would need to adjust your serving size of protein powder to just 24 grams or so) and 12 oz of banana.

APPENDIX B: FOOD JOURNAL AND DIET SAMPLES

BREAKFAST	COMPLEX CARB	PROTEIN SOURCE	FATS
TIME:			**SUPPLEMENTS** ☐ Multiple vitamin/mineral ☐ Chromium picolinate (200 mcg) ☐ Vitamin C (1000 mg)

SNACK	SIMPLE CARB	PROTEIN SOURCE	FATS
TIME:			**SUPPLEMENTS** ☐ Protein powder or meal replacement if no real food is consumed

LUNCH	COMPLEX CARB	PROTEIN SOURCE	FATS
TIME:			**SUPPLEMENTS** ☐ Vitamin C (1000 mg)

SNACK	SIMPLE CARB	PROTEIN SOURCE	FATS
TIME:			**SUPPLEMENTS** ☐Protein powder or meal replacement if no real food is consumed

DINNER	COMPLEX CARB	PROTEIN SOURCE	FATS
TIME:			**SUPPLEMENTS** ☐Vitamin C (1000 mg) ☐Creatine Monohydrate (2.5-3 grams)-Optional

POST WORKOUT	SIMPLE CARB	PROTEIN SOURCE	FATS
TIME:			**SUPPLEMENTS** ☐Protein powder or meal replacement if no real food is consumed ☐Creatine monohydrate (2.5–3 grams)—optional ☐L-Glutamine (5–10 grams)—optional

HARDGAINERS

Protein Shake Recipes

While this is by no means a full list of all of the combinations of things that can be done with protein and meal replacement powders, it is a list of my favorite ones that I have tries at one time or another.

CINNAMON OATMEAL BREAKFAST

Cook 1 cup of old fashioned oats. Let cool down for 5 minutes or so. Add some water and mix a packet of Prolab's Cinnamon Oatmeal Lean Mass Matrix.

Calories: Approximately 700
Carbohydrates: 94 grams
Protein: 50 grams
Fats: 13 grams

STRAWBERRY/BANANA SMOOTHIE

Add 2 cups of fresh strawberries and 2 eight-ounce bananas to 16 ounces of skim milk in a blender. Then add 1-1/2 scoop of vanilla whey protein such a Beverly's Muscle Provider or Prolab's Pure Whey. Add 1 tablespoon of flaxseed oil, some ice cubes to the mix and blend for 30 seconds on high speed to a minute. Then serve and enjoy!

Calories: Approximately 734
Carbohydrates: 98 grams
Protein: 54 grams
Fats: 14 grams
NOTE: Can also use chocolate powder as well.

CHOCOLATE/PEANUT BUTTER DELIGHT

Add 1 packet of Prolab's chocolate lean mass matrix to 16 ounces of skim milk on a blender. Then add 2 tablespoons of natural old fashioned peanut butter, some ice cubes to the mix and blend for 30 seconds on high speed to a minute. Then serve and enjoy!

Calories: Approximately 696
Carbohydrates: 60 grams
Protein: 60 grams
Fats: 24 grams

APPLE PIE SMOOTHIE

Blend 1 apple, 1 six-ounce banana, 1 teaspoon of cinnamon, and 1 vanilla meal replacement of your choice (I use Lean Mass Matrix most of the time) in 20 ounces of skim milk. Add some ice cubes to the mix and blend for 30 seconds on high speed to a minute.

Calories: Approximately 696
Carbohydrates: 704 grams
Protein: 58 grams
Fats: 8 grams

N-LARGE 2 LEMON SMOOTHIE

Blend 3 scoops of Prolab's vanilla N-Large 2 powder in 16 ounces of skim milk. Add 7 lemons and some ice cubes to the mix and blend for 30 seconds on high speed to a minute.

Calories: Approximately 758
Carbohydrates: 119 grams
Protein: 57 grams
Fats: 6 grams

N-LARGE 2 STRAWBERRY/CHERRIES SMOOTHIE

Blend 3 scoops of Prolab's strawberry N-Large 2

powder in 16 ounces of skim milk. Add 1 cup of cherries and some ice cubes to the mix and blend for 30 seconds on high speed to a minute.

Calories: Approximately 750
Carbohydrates: 114 grams
Protein: 57 grams
Fats: 6 grams

N-LARGE 2 ORANGE SMOOTHIE

Blend 3 scoops of Prolab's vanilla N-Large 2 powder in 16 ounces of skim milk. Add 2 oranges and some ice cubes to the mix and blend for 30 seconds on high speed to a minute.

Calories: Approximately 770
Carbohydrates: 122 grams
Protein: 57 grams
Fats: 6 grams

Appendix C: Break-In Routine

The routine recommended in this book is designed for athletes who have been weight training for at least 5 months consistently. If you are new to weight training (or follow a routine that is far less intensive than the routine recommended here), you need to first follow these pre-conditioning steps designed to prepare the body for what is to come and avoid injuries. Since you are new to weight training, you will get amazing results from this routine. Skipping this phase will result in you getting excessively sore and not reaping the benefits of the advanced routine. (Note: Even if you use this routine instead of the advanced routine, it is still necessary to follow the rules for anabolic nutrition in Chapter 3).

WEEKS: 1—4
DURATION: 4 WEEKS

MONDAY/THURSDAY				FULL BODY
EXERCISE	**PAGE NO.**	**REPS**	**SETS**	**REST**
MODIFIED COMPOUND SUPERSET				
(Rest 1 minute after the 1st set of exercise #1, and then do the first set of exercise #2. Rest a minute and go back to exercise #1. Continue this pattern until both exercises are done for the prescribed amount of sets).				
Dumbbell Bench Press	76	10	2	1 minute
Pull-down to Front (wide grip)	94	10	2	1 minute
MODIFIED COMPOUND SUPERSET				
Bent-over Lateral Raises	122	10	2	1 minute
Dumbbell Shoulder Press	116	10	2	1 minute
MODIFIED COMPOUND SUPERSET				
Incline Dumbbell Curls	140	10	2	1 minute
Overhead Dumbbell Triceps Extensions	164	10	2	1 minute
MODIFIED COMPOUND SUPERSET				
Leg Extensions	182	10	2	1 minute
Lying Leg Curls	204	10	2	1 minute
Squats	177	10	2	1 minute
Standing Calf Raises	218	10	2	1 minute
SUPERSET				
Lying Leg Raises	240	13-15	2	No Rest
Crunches	238	13-15	2	1 minute

Break-In Routine

WEEKS: 4—8

DURATION: 4 WEEKS

MONDAY/WEDNESDAY/FRIDAY				FULL BODY
EXERCISE	**PAGE NO.**	**REPS**	**SETS**	**REST**
MODIFIED COMPOUND SUPERSET				
(Rest 1 minute after the 1st set of exercise 1 and then do the first set of exercise 2. Rest a minute and go back to exercise 1. Continue this pattern until both exercises are done for the prescribed amount of sets).				
Incline Dumbbell Press	74	10	2	1 minute
One Arm Dumbbell Rows	96	10	2	1 minute
MODIFIED COMPOUND SUPERSET				
Dumbbell Bench Press	76	10	2	1 minute
Pull-down to Front (wide grip)	94	10	2	1 minute
MODIFIED COMPOUND SUPERSET				
Bent-over Lateral Raises	122	10	2	1 minute
Dumbbell Shoulder Press	116	10	2	1 minute
MODIFIED COMPOUND SUPERSET				
Incline Dumbbell Curls	140	10	2	1 minute
Overhead Dumbbell Triceps Extensions	164	10	2	1 minute
MODIFIED COMPOUND SUPERSET				
Leg Extensions	182	10	2	1 minute
Lying Leg Curls	204	10	2	1 minute
Squats	177	10	2	1 minute
Standing Calf Raises	218	10	2	1 minute
SUPERSET				
Lying Leg Raises	240	13-15	2	No Rest
Crunches	238	13-15	2	1 minute

HARDGAINERS

Break-In Routine
WEEKS: 9–12
DURATION: 4 WEEKS

MONDAY/THURSDAY				FULL BODY
EXERCISE	PAGE NO.	REPS	SETS	REST
MODIFIED COMPOUND SUPERSET				
(Rest 1 minute after the 1st set of exercise1 and then do the first set of exercise 2. Rest a minute and go back to exercise 1. Continue this pattern until both exercises are done for the prescribed amount of sets).				
Incline Dumbbell Press	74	10	3	1 minute
One Arm Dumbbell Rows	96	10	3	1 minute
MODIFIED COMPOUND SUPERSET				
Dumbbell Bench Press	76	10	3	1 minute
Pull-down to Front (wide grip)	94	10	3	1 minute
MODIFIED COMPOUND SUPERSET				
Bent-over Lateral Raises	122	10	3	1 minute
Dumbbell Shoulder Press	116	10	3	1 minute
MODIFIED COMPOUND SUPERSET				
Incline Dumbbell Curls	140	10	3	1 minute
Overhead Dumbbell Triceps Extensions	164	10	3	1 minute
MODIFIED COMPOUND SUPERSET				
Leg Extensions	182	10	2	1 minute
Lying Leg Curls	204	10	2	1 minute
Squats	177	10	2	1 minute
Standing Calf Raises	218	10	2	1 minute
SUPERSET				
Lying Leg Raises	240	13-15	2	No Rest
Crunches	238	13-15	2	1 minute

Break-In Routine

WEEKS: 9–12

DURATION: 4 WEEKS

TUESDAY/FRIDAY				FULL BODY
EXERCISE	**PAGE NO.**	**REPS**	**SETS**	**REST**
MODIFIED COMPOUND SUPERSET				
Squats	177	10	3	1 minute
Lying Leg Curls	204	10	3	1 minute
MODIFIED COMPOUND SUPERSET				
Leg Extensions	182	10	3	1 minute
Dumbbell Stiff-Legged Deadlifts	200	10	3	1 minute
MODIFIED COMPOUND SUPERSET				
Standing Calf Raises	218	10	3	1 minute
Seated Calf Raises	224	10-20	3	1 minute
MODIFIED COMPOUND SUPERSET				
Lying Leg Raises	240	13-15	3	1 minutes
Crunches	238	13-15	3	1 minute

Break-In Routine
WEEKS: 13–16
DURATION: 3 WEEKS

MONDAY/THURSDAY				FULL BODY
EXERCISE	**PAGE NO.**	**REPS**	**SETS**	**REST**
SUPERSET				
Incline Dumbbell Press	74	10	3	no rest
One Arm Dumbbell Rows	96	10	3	1 minute
SUPERSET				
Dumbbell Bench Press	76	10	3	no rest
Pulldown to Front (wide grip)	94	10	3	1 minute
MODIFIED COMPOUND SUPERSET				
Bent-over Lateral Raises	122	10	3	no rest
Dumbbell Shoulder Press	116	10	3	1 minute
MODIFIED COMPOUND SUPERSET				
Incline Dumbbell Curls	140	10	3	no rest
Overhead Dumbbell Triceps Extensions	164	10	3	1 minute

TUESDAY/FRIDAY				FULL BODY
EXERCISE	**PAGE NO.**	**REPS**	**SETS**	**REST**
SUPERSET				
Squats	177	10	3	no rest
Lying Leg Curls	204	10	3	1 minute
SUPERSET				
Leg Extensions	182	10	3	no rest
Dumbbell Stiff-Legged Deadlifts	200	10	3	1 minute
MODIFIED COMPOUND SUPERSET				
Standing Calf Raises	218	10	3	no rest
Seated Calf Raise	224	10-20	3	1 minute
MODIFIED COMPOUND SUPERSET				
Lying Leg Raises	240	13-15	3	no rest
Crunches	238	13-15	3	1 minute

Break-In Routine

WEEKS: 17–20

DURATION: 3 WEEKS

MONDAY/THURSDAY				FULL BODY
EXERCISE	**PAGE NO.**	**REPS**	**SETS**	**REST**
SUPERSET				
Incline Dumbbell Press	74	10	4	no rest
One Arm Dumbbell Rows	96	10	4	1 minute
SUPERSET				
Dumbbell Bench Press	76	10	3	no rest
Pull-down to Front (wide grip)	94	10	3	1 minute
MODIFIED COMPOUND SUPERSET				
Bent-over Lateral Raises	122	10	3	no rest
Dumbbell Shoulder Press	116	10	3	1 minute
MODIFIED COMPOUND SUPERSET				
Incline Dumbbell Curls	140	10	4	no rest
Overhead Dumbbell Triceps Extensions	164	10	4	1 minute

TUESDAY/FRIDAY				FULL BODY
EXERCISE	**PAGE NO.**	**REPS**	**SETS**	**REST**
SUPERSET				
Squats	177	10	4	no rest
Lying Leg Curls	204	10	4	1 minute
SUPERSET				
Leg Extensions	182	10	3	no rest
Dumbbell Stiff-Legged Deadlifts	200	10	3	1 minute
MODIFIED COMPOUND SUPERSET				
Standing Calf Raises	218	10	4	no rest
Seated Calf Raise	224	10-20	4	1 minute
MODIFIED COMPOUND SUPERSET				
Lying Leg Raises	240	13-15	3	no rest
Crunches	238	13-15	3	1 minute

APPENDIX D: FURTHER INFORMATION ABOUT CREATINE

CREATINE CYCLING

Another point to talk about is the issue of cycling (or cessation of use) of the supplement creatine. If creatine was a supplement that loses its effectiveness as time goes by then I would recommend cycling. For example, it is beneficial to cycle fat burning supplements containing caffeine and ephedrine as the body's receptors begin to attenuate after 2 to 3 weeks of continual use. Once the body gets used to them, you need to either increase the dosage or stop their use so that the body begins to respond once again. However, that is not the way that creatine works. Basically, creatine gets stored into your muscles and you get the effects mentioned above, period. It is really straightforward. As far as the initial weight gain that you may experience when you start taking it is concerned, whether you cycle it or not, you will get the same amount of initial weight gain as that extra weight is determined by the amount of intracellular fluid retention that your muscle cells can store (something that remains static). The reason I say "the weight gain that you may experience" is because sometimes the scale does not register any weight gain. For instance, if you increase the sets and repitions in your workout while keeping calories the same, you may lose fat as you gain added muscle volume. However, the lack of weight gain by the scale does not mean that you are not responding to the creatine. To gauge creatine's efficacy on you, judge it by the muscle appearance effects and the performance enhancement in the gym.

SIDE EFFECTS

The only adverse side effect that I have experienced in my more than two years of continual use is the gastric upset at the beginning of use. After a couple of weeks or so my system adapted to absorbing the powder. Other than that, I have not observed any other side effects. Keep in mind, however, that the liver and kidneys have to process this compound. Therefore, I would not recommend it for someone with kidney problems or liver problems. Also, even if you are completely healthy ensure more than adequate hydration levels (body weight x 0.66 = total ounces of water to drink per day) and if you drink coffee, add an extra 16 ounces of water for every cup that you drink over the day.

A side effect that I have read about but I am unable to verify is that your body's production of creatine shuts down. However, after cessation of use, according to all of the literature your body's production kicks in again. No adverse effects have been documented due to the creatine shutdown created by the body.

WHAT HAPPENS IF I STOP TAKING IT

After two weeks your creatine levels go back to normal. You will also feel weaker for about 3 weeks because your ATP system is no longer enhanced. You'll also lose your enhanced recovery capabilities. In this sense, and only in this sense, creatine is kind of like steroids. The difference is that creatine can be taken safely all of the time (personal opinion) while with steroids you already know the story.

However, in creatine's defense, I can also say that creatine is no different than weight training. What happens if you stop going to the gym? Will you look the same three months later?

Seriously speaking, however, since you already were lifting heavier weights while using the compound, your nervous system will remember those weights and you will be able to get back to them after 3 to 6 weeks. However, I would lower the volume if I were coming off it.

Creatine and Caffeine Intake

Years ago there were some studies suggesting that the effects of creatine were cancelled if you also had caffeine. For people like me that most of the time keep caffeine at bay this does not pose any problems. However, this is not the case for people on fat-burning formulas that contain it. While I don't use the amount of water that the caffeine users in the study were taking, the training protocol, or any other testing parameters, my recommendation is that you take the caffeine (or the fat burning supplement) at a time separate from your creatine intake (i.e. take your creatine after the workout with your protein shake and take your fat burner before the workout). Also, be sure that you follow the hydration guidelines described above.

Carbohydrate-Laden Creatine

Due to studies out there demonstrating that the body's uptake of creatine is greater when you take it with carbs, most companies out there have been creating products that contain creatine but also high levels of sugar. My advice to you is: save your money. Buy the powder form instead as you will get many more servings of the pure compound. As long as you take it after the workout with a protein/carbohydrate-rich shake I guarantee that your body will absorb the creatine with the utmost efficiency.

Conclusions

In my view, the greatest advantage that creatine gives you (besides the cosmetic effect of bigger and fuller muscles) is that it enables you to handle more volume and recover faster in between sets by upgrading the body's capabilities to produce ATP, thereby decreasing the production of lactic acid. Therefore, in my opinion, people that will get the most benefit from creatine are those that follow a high volume, short rest in between sets type of workout. Remember that the more work that you can cram into an hour the more you'll grow (if you cycle volume and intensity as we discussed in previous articles).

Again, as I have said in previous articles, even though I believe that creatine is a safe supplement, don't take my word for it if you have doubts. Do your own research and objectively review the data. If you feel creatine may be good for you, then just follow the recommendations laid out in this article and provided your overall training and nutrition strategy are good, I guarantee that you will see results from it.

APPENDIX E: GLOSSARY OF TERMS

Aerobic Exercise: Constant moderate intensity work that uses up oxygen at a rate at which the cardiorespiratory system can replenish oxygen in the working muscles. Examples of such activity are stationary bike riding or walking. It is a good activity for fat loss when done in the right amounts but highly catabolic if done in excess.

Anaerobic Exercise: Exercise in which oxygen is used up more quickly than the body is able to replenish it inside the working muscle. Weight training is an example of such an activity. It is highly anabolic in nature but also highly catabolic if done in excess.

Anabolic State: Favorable state in the body created by a combination of good training, nutrition, and rest that leads to favorable changes in body composition.

Anabolic Steroids: Synthetic (human-made) hormones that simulate the effects of the male hormone testosterone.

Anti-catabolic Properties: Properties provided by certain nutrients that protect the muscle mass in the body from being broken down.

Anti-lypolitic Properties: Properties provided by certain nutrients that prevent the body from turning calories into fat.

Antioxidant Properties: Properties provided by certain nutrients that protect the body from disease.

Basic Exercises: Exercise movement that involves a large number of muscles in the body. They are generally multi-joint movements that target the larger muscles of the body (such as chest, back, and thighs) but also involve the smaller muscles as well (such as shoulders, arms, calves, and abs) as auxiliary muscles. Examples of such movements are chin-ups, pull-ups, dips, bench presses, squats, and lunges.

Biological Value (BV) of a Protein: Value that measures how well the body can absorb and utilize a protein. The higher the biological value of the protein you use, the more nitrogen your body can absorb, use, and retain. As a result, proteins with the highest BV promote the most lean muscle gains. Whey protein has the highest BV value, rating 104. Egg protein is only second to whey rating, a 100 with milk proteins being a close third rating as 91. Beef rates 80 with soy proteins a distant 74. Bean proteins, due to the fact that they are plant-based proteins, only rate 49.

Bulk Minerals: Minerals that the body needs in great quantities (in the order of grams) such as calcium, magnesium, potassium, sodium and phosphorus.

Carbohydrates: Macronutrient used by the body as its main source of energy. Carbohydrates are divided into complex carbs and simple carbs. The complex carbs give you sustained energy ("timed release") while the simple carbs gives you immediate energy. This macronutrient can be found in rice (complex, starchy), pasta (complex, starchy), breads (complex, starchy), fruits (simple), sugars (simple), fruit juices (simple), dairy products (simple), and vegetables (complex, fibrous).

Catabolic State: Unfavorable state in the body created by a combination of too much training, lack of good nutrition, and lack of rest that leads to muscle loss and fat accumulation.

Concentric Movement: Portion of the exercise where the muscle contracts. This happens when you are lifting the weight. This portion of the movement should be performed as fast as possible (once you are past the beginner period) without involving momentum.
Beginners should concentrate, however, on performing the movement slowly and deliberately.

Cortisol: Catabolic hormone secreted by the adrenal glands in situations of stress (both physical and mental), lack of calories/nutrients and lack of sleep. This hormone is associated with loss of muscle mass, loss of strength, and fat accumulation. An excess of it over long periods of time may also contribute to hardening of the arteries; something that leads to heart disease.

Diuretics: Drugs used to remove excess water from the body. There are two versions: the drug version (can only be prescribed by a physician), and the herbal version. Excessive use of the drug version has as side effects muscle cramps and harsh arrhythmia. The herbal version, while safer than the drug version, can lead to potassium loss and excessive use puts stress on the kidneys.

Dumbbell: A short-handled barbell 10-12 inches long that can be carried in one hand. Dumbbells allow for flexibility in the execution of a movement and for full range of motion.

Eccentric Movement: Portion of the movement in which the muscle elongates. This happens as you lower the weight back to the starting position. This portion of the movement should be performed slowly and deliberately.

Endorphins: Hormones that make us feel good and happy. The production of these hormones is stimulated by exercise.

Essential Fatty Acids (EFAs): Fats that have anti-catabolic, anti-lypolitic, and antioxidant properties. These fats affect the good cholesterol in a positive way. In addition, these fats aid in the muscle-building, fat-loss process. The omega-3 fatty acids found in fats such as fish oils and flaxseed oil are a good source of EFAs.

Estrogen: Female hormone that regulates and sustains female sexual development and reproductive function. An excess of this hormone appears to be related to heart disease and cancer.

In addition, when this hormone is in excess, it causes fat gain and water retention. Estrogen deficits, on the other hand, include memory problems, trouble finding words, inability to pay attention, mood swings, and irritability. By helping to balance the levels of this hormone, exercise helps reduce the risk of these diseases and conditions.

Exercise Volume: The amount of work performed in an exercise session defined by the product resulting from the amount of weight lifted, multiplied by the number of sets and multiplied by the number of repetitions. For example, if you had a workout that consisted of 10 sets of dumbbell curls, and for each set you used 30 pounds and performed 10 repetitions, then your biceps routine volume equals 10 x 10 x 30 = 3000 pounds. Too much volume leads to overtraining.

Fats: Macronutrient needed by the body in order to manufacture hormones and sustain cell metabolism. All the cells in the body have some fat in them. Hormones are manufactured from fats. Also, fats lubricate your joints. If you eliminate the fat from your diet, your hormonal production will go down and a whole array of chemical reactions will be interrupted. There are three types of fats: saturated, polyunsaturated and monounsaturated.

Fat Soluble Vitamins: Vitamins that get stored in fat that if taken in excessive amounts will become toxic. They include vitamins A, D, E, and K.

Giant Set: Giant Sets are 4 exercises done one after the other with no rest in between sets. Again, there are two ways to implement this. You can either use 4 exercises for the same muscle group or perform 2 pairs of opposing muscle group exercises. For the purposes of this manual, whenever we do giant sets, we will perform two pairs of opposing muscle group exercises with no rest. The exception is when we do abs in which we will alternate between lower abs and upper abs.

Growth Hormone: Hormone secreted by the pituitary gland that aids in fat loss and muscle building.

Hormones: Fats similar to, and usually synthesized from, cholesterol, starting with acetyl-CoA, moving through squalene, past lanosterol, into cholesterol, and, in the gonads and adrenal cortex, back to a number of steroid hormones. Because they stimulate cell growth, either by changing the internal structure or increasing the rate of proliferation, they are often called anabolic steroids.

Hypertrophy: Scientific term for describing an increase in muscle mass and strength caused by the stimulation of the muscles.

Intensity: Intensity has two definitions in the weight-training world. (1) Relative term that indicates the level of effort exerted during the performance of an exercise. (2) In the strength training circles, intensity refers to the amount of weight being used on a specific exercise.

Insulin: Hormone secreted by the pancreas responsible for carbohydrate metabolism. This hormone determines if the carbohydrates are to be used for energy, for storage inside the muscle cells as glycogen, or for converting and storing the carbohydrates as fats when they are found in excess in the bloodstream.

Isolation Exercises: Exercise movements that are generally single-jointed and serve to isolate a single area of the body. Examples of such are dumbbell flies, concentration curls, triceps kickbacks, leg extensions, and leg curls.

Lactic Acid: Byproduct created by a lack of oxygen flow to the working muscles. Lactic acid is created by anaerobic activities such as weight training exercises. It is believed that its presence causes a surge in growth hormone levels.

Macronutrient: One of the three major nutrients that the body needs for survival. These nutrients are carbohydrates, proteins, and fats.

Metabolism: The rate at which the body utilizes calories and nutrients in order to sustain its daily activities.

Minerals: Minerals are inorganic compounds (not produced by animals or vegetables) whose main function is to assure that your brain receives the correct signals from the body, as well as to ensure balance of fluids, make muscular contractions possible, and allow energy production, as well as

the building of muscle and bones. There are two types of minerals: bulk and trace minerals.

Modified Compound Superset: In a modified compound set, you pair exercises for opposing muscle groups or for opposing muscle movements (e.g. push vs. pull). First you perform one exercise, rest the recommended amount of seconds and then perform the second exercise (for instance, first do biceps, rest, then do triceps). You then rest the prescribed amount of time again and go back to the first exercise. Using this technique of pairing exercises in a modified superset fashion not only saves time and keeps the body warm, but also allows for faster recovery of the nervous system between sets. This will allow the person to lift heavier weights than possible if he just stayed idle for 2 to 3 minutes waiting to recover.

Monounsaturated Fats: Fats that have a positive effect on the good cholesterol levels. These fats are usually high in the essential fatty acids and may have antioxidant properties. Sources of these fats are fish oils, virgin olive oil, canola oil, and flaxseed oil.

Muscle Failure: Point during the exercise at which it becomes impossible to perform another repetition in good form. This point is reached due to the lack of oxygen reaching the working muscles and the increased levels of lactic acid.

Neutral Grip: A grip on a parallel bar that allows your palms to be facing each other. In this grip, your thumbs are pointing up. For example, a low pulley row with the traditional V-bar is an exercise that uses a neutral grip. Chest dips on parallel bars also use a neutral grip.

Overtraining: Condition caused by an excess of volume in a training routine that leads to muscle loss, strength loss, and fat accumulation. Symptoms include depression, insomnia, lethargy, and lack of energy.

Polyunsaturated Fats: Fats that do not have an effect in cholesterol levels. Most of the fats in vegetable oils, such as corn, cottonseed, safflower, soybean, and sunflower oil are polyunsaturated.

Pronated Grip: a grip on the bar when your palms are facing down and away from you. In this grip your thumbs are pointing inward to each other. For example, a close-grip pulldown to front is an exercise that uses a pronated grip.

Protein: Every tissue in your body is made from protein (i.e. muscle, hair, skin, nails). Proteins are the building blocks of muscle tissue. This macronutrient can be found in poultry, meats, and dairy products.

Repetitions: The number of times that you perform an exercise. For instance, pretend that you are performing a bench press. You pick up the bar, you lower it, pause and lift it up. That action of executing the movement for one time counts for one repetition. If you perform that same move-

ment a second time, then that is your second repetition, and so on.

Rest Interval: The amount of time that a person rests in between sets. For instance, a rest interval of 60 seconds means that after you finish your first set, you will remain idle for 60 seconds before going on to the next set.

Saturated Fats: Saturated fats are associated with heart disease and high cholesterol levels. They are found to a large extent in products of animal origin. However, some vegetable fats are altered in a way that increases the amount of saturated fats in them by a chemical process known as hydrogenation. Hydrogenated vegetable oils are generally found in packaged foods. In addition, coconut oil, palm oil, and palm kernel oil, which are also frequently used in packaged foods, and non-dairy creamers are also highly saturated.

Sets: A set is a collection of repetitions that culminates in the muscle reaching muscular failure. Muscular failure is the point at which, due to a buildup of lactic acid in the muscle, it becomes impossible to perform another repetition with good form.

Supersets: A superset is a combination of one exercises performed one right after the other with no rest in between. There are two ways to implement a superset. The first way is to do two exercises for the same muscle group at once; like doing dumbbell curls immediately followed by concentration curls. The drawback to this technique is that you will not be as strong as you usually are on the second exercise. The second and best way to superset is by pairing exercises of opposing muscle groups or different muscle movements such as back and chest, thighs and hamstrings, biceps and triceps, shoulders and calves, upper abs and lower abs. When pairing antagonistic exercises, there is no drop of strength whatsoever once your cardiovascular system is well conditioned.

Supinated Grip: A grip on the bar in which your palms are facing up toward you. This is most commonly known as a reverse grip. In this grip, your thumbs are pointing outward and away from each other. For example, a close-grip chin using a reverse grip (palms up) is an exercise that uses a supinated grip.

Trace Minerals: Minerals that are needed by the body in minute amounts, usually of micrograms, such as chromium, copper, cobalt, silicon, selenium, iron, and zinc.

Testosterone: Hormone responsible for increasing muscle size. Even though this hormone is predominantly present in males, it is also present in females to a lesser degree. It is believed that this hormone also aids in fat loss to a lesser degree.

Vitamins: Vitamins are organic compounds (produced by both animals and vegetables) whose function is to enhance the actions of proteins that cause chemical reactions such as muscle building, fat burning and energy production. There are two types of vitamins: fat-soluble and water-soluble.

Water Soluble Vitamins: Vitamins that are not stored in the body, such as the B-complex vitamins and vitamin C. Therefore, they need to be taken on a frequent basis.

APPENDIX F: WEBSITES AND REFERENCES

USEFUL WEBSITES

www.Hardgainers.net

Visit this website for free downloads for hardgainer's training and nutrition charts as well as to get your questions from the book answered.

www.HRFit.net

A visit here will reward you with a well-rounded bushel of information written by Hugo Rivera, ranging from how to design a workout routine to whether to select or reject a food supplement. If you have a question on fitness it will most likely be answered here.

www.BodyTechOnline.com

The home of bodybuilding coach and guru Tim Gardner who owns the finest 12,000 sq. ft health and fitness club in the Tampa Bay area called BODY* TECH Fitness Emporium. BODY*TECH offers a full size weight training area, cardio deck, personal training staff, massage therapist, BODY*TECH cafe, tanning beds, pro shop, personalized diets, and day care. If you are ever around here in Florida in this neck of the woods, Tim's place is the one to go to. Tim Gardner, who has gotten in shape hundreds of athletes for their respective competitions, also offers discounted supplements/products through his website as well as diet/training design services, contest preparation advice for bodybuilding, fitness or figure shows, and training DVDs.

www.GetFitNow.com

A powerful resource for anyone seeking advice, knowledge, and more. Loaded with news, fitness tips, and discussion forums, this is a must see.

www.Getfitzone.com

Renaissance Health & Fitness is an exclusive health and fitness personal training studio for men and women of all ages located in Tierra Verde Florida. Owned by fitness expert Andre Hudson, the studio features a wide selection of the latest resistance training and cardiovascular equipment, qualified personal trainers and many additional amenities to make your workout enjoyable. Whether you need to lose, gain, or simply improve your overall conditioning, Andre Hudson's Renaissance Health & Fitness has everything you need to help you to achieve your goals!

www.Bodybuilding.com

Tons of free information on anything you need to know about bodybuilding and fitness written by several experts in the industry. They also carry most supplement brands in the market, selling them at a huge discount. Their customer service is second to none as well, so when you place an order you get it within a few days.

www.Powerblocks.com

Home of the PowerBlocks, here you will find the world's most efficient dumbbells in terms of space and feasibility of changing the weights.

www.IronMaster.com

Home of the Quick-Lock Dumbbells, here you find the most economical, sturdy, and safe set of adjustable dumbbells anywhere.

www.FitnessFactory.com

Great place to fulfill your home gym equipment needs. They have awesome customer service and great prices.

www.Prolab.com

Homepage of my favorite line of supplements. I was using Prolab products long before they took me in as a sponsored athlete back in 2002. I have always liked Prolab as they carry all of the basic supplements that bodybuilders need. In addition, all of their supplements are produced with state-of-the-art manufacturing and also sold at the right price. Back in the days when creatine was super expensive, Prolab was distributing the super-pure German-grade creatine in buy one, get one free twinpack bottles. Hard to compete with good quality at an attractive price.

www.InfinityFitness.com

Website of training and nutrition consultant Scott Mendelsohn. Scott is a super awesome and knowledgeable guy who has tons of free information on his site written by himself and doctors that are experts in nutrition. He also carries state of the art products as well.

www.DaveDraper.com

Dave is a bodybuilding legend whom I am most grateful to know and be able to call a friend. My first articles, as a matter of fact, were published on his site back in 1999. Winner of Mr. America, Mr. World and Mr. Universe, Dave shares his extensive knowledge in a very straightforward, simple, and almost poetic manner. The man is a wealth of knowledge and those who visit his site will greatly benefit from it.

www.MuscleBuildingDiet.com

Owned by Todd Mendelsohn, a former Mr. Central Florida who works as a nutrition/training consultant. If you want more advanced tailor-made programs for bulking up, then this is the place to go. With his programs (and a lot of pain) I was able to put over 3 inches on my quadriceps, which used to be my weak body part. He is the one that you go to after you have mastered everything contained in this book, especially if future plans for competition are in your mind. Don't expect him to be easy though. He is the most brutal trainer I have ever met, with an archive of off-the-wall training routines designed for shock and awe.

TRAINING REFERENCES

Bompa, Tudor O. 1983. *Theory and Methodology of Training--The Key to Athletic Performance.* Kendall/ Hunt Publishing; Dubuque, Ia.

Bompa, Tudor O., Cornacchia, Lorenzo J. 1998. *Serious Strength Training.* Human Kinetics Publishers.

Bompa, Tudor O. 1990. "Periodization of Strength: The Most Effective Methodology of Strength Training." *National Strength and Conditioning Association Journal*, 12(5), 49-52.

Bompa, Tudor O. *Periodization of Strength: the New Wave in Strength Training*. Toronto, ON: Veritas Publishing Inc., pg. 28, 1993.

Chernyak, A.V., Karimov, E.S. Butinchinov, Z.T. 1979. "Distribution of Load Volume and Intensity Throughout the Year (Weightlifting)." *Soviet Sports Review*. 14(2): 98-101.

Ebbing, C. and P. Clarkson, 1989. "Exercise-Induced Muscle Damage and Adaptation." *Sports Medicine*. Vol 7: 207-234.

Edgerton, R.V. 1976. "Neuromuscular Adaptation. to Power and Endurance work." *Canadian Journal of Applied Sports Sciences*, 1:49–58.

Fleck, S.J. "Periodized Strength Training: A Critical Review." *The Journal of Strength and Conditioning Research*, 13 (1) 82-89, 1999.

Fry, A.C., Kreamer W.J., Stone, M.H., 2000. "Relationship Between Serum Testosterone, Cortisol, and Weightlifting Performance." *Journal of Strength and Conditioning Research*, 14(13): 338-343.

Fry, R.W., R. Morton, and D. Keast, 1991. "Overtraining in Athletics." *Sports Medicine*, 2(1):32-65.

Gilliam, G.M., 1981. "Effects of Frequency of Weight Training on Muscle Strength Training." *Journal of Sports Medicine*, 21: 432-436.

Goldberg, A.L., J.D.Etlinger,D.F.Goldspink, and C. Jablecki., 1975. "Mechanism of Work-Induced Hypertrophy of Skeletal Muscles." *Medicine and Science in Sports and Exercise*, 7:185-198.

Hakkinen, K., 1989. "Neuromuscular and Hormonal Adaptations During Strength and Power Training." *A Review of Sports Medicine Physical Fitness* 29(1):9-26.

Hakkinen K.A., A. Pskarinen, M. Alen, H. Kauhanen, P.V. Komi, 1987. "Relationships Between Training Volume, Physical Performance Capacity, and Serum Hormone Concentrations During Prolonged Training in Elite Weight Lifters." *International Journal of Sports Medicine*, 8 (suppli): 61-65.

Kuipers, H. and H.A. Keizer., 1988. "Overtraining in Elite Athletes: Review and Directions for the Future." *Sports Medicine*, 6:79-92.

McDonagh, M.J.N. and C.T.M. Davis, 1984. "Adaptive Response of Mammalian Skeletal Muscle to Exercise with High Loads." *European Journal of Applied Physiology*, 52:139-155.

Minchenko, V.G. 1989. "The Distribution of Training Load Throughout the Yearly Training Cycles of Athletes." *Soviet Sports Review*, 24(1): 1-6.

Rhea M.R., Ball S.D., Phillips W.T., Burkett L.N., 2002. "A Comparison of Linear and Daily Undulating Periodized Programs with equated Volume and Intensity for Strength." *J. Strength Cond. Res.* May;16(2):250-5.

Starkey, D.B., M.L., Pollock, Y., Ishida, Welsch, M.A., Brechue, W.F., Graves, J.E., Feigenbaum, M.S. 1996. "Effect of resistance training volume on strength and muscle thickness." *Medicine and Science in Sports and Exercise*, 1311–1320.

Terjung R.L., D.A. Hood, 1986. "Biochemical Adaptation in Skeletal Muscle Induced by Exercise Training." *Nutrition and Aerobic Exercise*, Am. Chem. Soc., 8–27.

NUTRITION REFERENCES
Dragan GI, Vasiliu A, Georgescu E., 1984. "Effects of Increased Supply of Protein on Elite Weightlifters." In *Milk Proteins*. Galesloot TE, Tinbergen BJ, (Eds). Pudoc, Wageningen, The Netherlands Pudoc, 99-103.

Ivy, J.L., 1991. "Muscle Glycogen Synthesis Before and After Exercise." *Sports Medicine*, 11:6-19.

emon, Peter W.R., 1991. "Protein and amino acid eeds of the strength athlete." *International ournal of Sports Nutrition*, 1:127-390.

nro, H.N., 1951. "Carbohydrate and fat as factor in protein utilization and metabolism." *Phys-Rev.*, 31:449-488.

STEROID REFERENCES
DiPasquale, M.G., 1990. *Anabolic Steroid Side Effects-Fact, Fiction and Treatment.* Warkworth, Ontario: MGD Press.

Lamb, D., 1984. "Anabolic steroids in athletics: how do they work and how dangerous are they?" *American Journal of Sports Medicine.* 12(1):31-37.

WHEY PROTEIN REFERENCES
Bounous, G., 1988. "Dietary whey protein inhibits the development of dimethylhydrazine induced malignancy." *Clin. Invest. Medic.* 213-217.

Bounous, G.P., Konshaven and P. Gold, 1988. "The Immuno-Enhancing Properties of Dietary Whey Protein Concentrates," *Clin. Invest. Med.* 11 271-278.

Burke, D.G. and P.D. Chilibeck, et al., 2001. "The Effect of Whey Protein Supplementation With and Without Creatne Monohydrate Combined With Resistance Training on Lean Tissue Mass and Muscle Strength," *Int. Jour. Sport Nutr. Exerc. Metab.* 11/3 349-64.

CREATINE REFERENCES
Odland, L.M., J.D. MacDougall, et al., 1997. "Effect of oral creatine supplementation on muscle [PCr] and short term maximum power output," *Med. Sci. Sports Exerc.* 29/2 p.216-9.

Pearson, D.R., D.G. Hamby, et al., 1999. "Long-term effects of creatine monohydrate on strength and power." *Journal of Strength and Conditioning*

Research 13/3 187-192.

Poortmans, J.R. and M. Francaux., 1999. "Long-term oral creatine supplementation does not impair renal function in healthy athletes" *Med. Sci. Sport. Exerc.* 31 1108-1110.

GLUTAMINE REFERENCES
Varnier, M. and G.P. Leese, et al., 1995. "Stimulatory effect of glutamine on glycogen accumulation in human skeletal muscle," *Am. Journal Physiol.* 269/2 pt. 1 E309-15.

Welbourne, T.C., 1995. "Increased Plasma Bicarbonate and Growth Hormone After an Oral Glutamine Load." *Am. Journal. Clin. Nutr.* 61/5 1058-61.

ANDROSTENEDIONE REFERENCES
King, D.S., et al., 1995.   "Effects of oral androstenedione on serum testosterone and adaptations to resistance training in young men," *JAMA* 281 2020-2028.

Rasmussen, B.B., et al., 1999. "Androstenedione does not stimulate muscle protein synthesis," *Jour. of FASEB* 13/4 (1999), p.546.

About the Author

Hugo A. Rivera, a University of South Florida graduate with a Bachelor of Science in Engineering and also a Trainer and Sports Nutrition Specialist certification from the ISSA, was born December 5, 1974 in Bayamon, Puerto Rico. As an overweight child he experienced at an early age the feelings of insecurity that come along with obesity as well as the scorn and ridicule from the people around him. After going anorexic at the age of 13 and losing a total of 70 pounds in less than a year, he was taken to a nutritionist by his concerned parents in an effort to stop the anorexic cycle. This nutritionist mentioned one thing that would change Hugo's outlook on dieting forever: "Eating food will not make you fat; only abusing the quantities of the bad foods will." After listening to that statement, Hugo decided to kick the anorexic habit and to dedicate his life to studying the effects of foods on the human physiology.

By the age of fifteen Hugo's interest in how food affects the shape and the form of your body naturally led to an interest in the area of exercise, something that led him to become an avid natural bodybuilder.

Discovering early on that there wasn't much realistic or practical bodybuilding or fitness advice, he went on to start recording what worked and what didn't for him. After much trial and error, he started finding principles that he noticed worked on any healthy human being. The best part of it all was his discovery on the fact that there was no necessity to stay all day at the gym in order to get results! Upset at the fact that not many people in the indus-

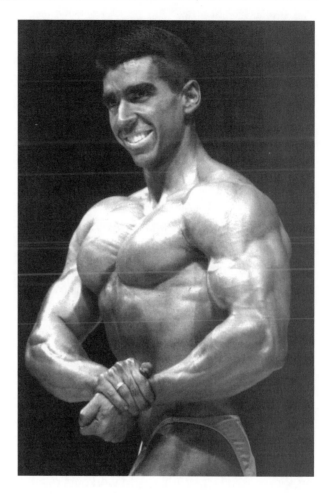

try cared about trainees actually reaching their goals, he decided to create a web site and start conducting personal training during his college years in an effort to spread all of the knowledge that he had acquired.

Fourteen years later Hugo holds a Statewide Natural Bodybuilding Title (Mr. Typhoon Bay) and also a 4th Place in the Welterweight Class of the Nationwide NPC Team Universe (the natural bodybuilder's highest and most competitive contest). Hugo is now considered an expert in the industry and he has dedicated much of his time to helping normal people achieve their dream figures by sharing sensible and practical knowledge that he has found over the years to work even on the most stubborn metabolisms. Hugo has shared his knowledge in his website www.hrfit.net, as well as on several articles published in Natural Muscle Magazine www.naturalmuscle.net, Olympian's Mind and Body News www.olympian.it, in online e-zines such as Dolfzine.com, www.davedraper.com, www.bodybuilding.com and www.bodybuilding.about.com amongst others. Also, Hugo authored a self-published bodybuilding manual called *Body Re-Engineering* along with two best selling books published by Hatherleigh Press targeted towards the weight loss community called *The Body Sculpting Bible for Men* and *The Body Sculpting Bible for Women* (featuring the 14 Day Body Sculpting Program). Hugo wrote these books in conjunction with James Villepigue, an authority in exercise form and the connection between the mind and the muscle. In these books, both authors apply the periodization principles used by pro athletes to workouts geared for people whose main goal is to lose weight and firm up. In addition, he co-authored nutrition and training programs along with nationally recognized fitness icon and six time Ms. Olympia Cory Everson. He has also served as consultant to nutrition companies in designing nutritional formulas and also currently represents Prolab Nutrition by going to several nutrition stores and educating the public on training, nutrition and supplementation with Prolab's products.

Hugo's knowledge of the human physiology and anatomy (something that he was exposed to from an early age due to the fact that his grandfather was a Medical Doctor), combined with his analytical skills that he developed in his engineering profession enable him to produce extremely efficient programs that anyone can fit on their schedule. The fact that he was overweight and then extremely underweight (after the anorexic period) enables him to identify with all groups of people that have weight problems. In addition, the fact that for many years he held a steady hectic engineering job in addition to his successful online and personal training business enables him to offer practical advice that all people who live a hectic lifestyle can follow.

PUBLISHED WORKS

Body Re-Engineering
The Body Sculpting Bible for Men
The Body Sculpting Bible for Women
The Body Sculpting Bible
  Express—Men's Edition
The Body Sculpting Bible
  Express—Women's Edition

CONTEST HISTORY

NPC 2001 Typhoon Bay
(Statewide Level Show)
Placing: Lightweight Champion
                Unanimous Overall Champion
NPC 2002 Team Universe
(National Level Show)
Placing: 4th Welterweight Champion
NPC 2004 National Bodybuilding
Championships (National Level Show)
Placing: 16th Middleweight

Get fit now with

HEALTHY · LIVING · BOOKS

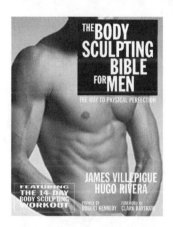

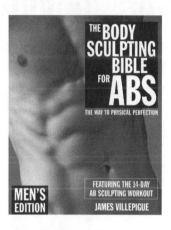

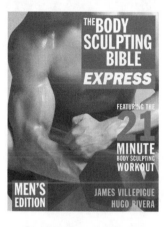

THE BODY SCULPTING BIBLE FOR MEN

The ultimate workout program for men who are looking for total body results.

"The most complete, effective fitness manual out there."
—**Musclemag International**

$17.95

ISBN 1-57826-085-X

THE BODY SCULPTING BIBLE FOR ABS

The definitive guide to sculpting rock-hard, chiseled abs.

$14.95

ISBN I-57826-I34-I

THE BODY SCULPTING BIBLE EXPRESS —MEN'S EDITION

Featuring the 21 Minute Body Sculpting Workout

From the experts that started the body sculpting phenomenon comes a revolutionary new workout designed to tone and chisel your body in just 21 minutes a day.

$15.95

ISBN I-57826-I84-8

Available at bookstores everywhere

(if you don't see it, ask for it) or call toll-free:

1-800-906-1234

Visit us on the web at **www.getfitnow.com**

Cut your workout time in half with Muscles in Minutes

The Insiders' Guide to Body Building with Negative Training

Now you can cut your workout time and increase your results with the revolutionary technique of "forced negatives" or eccentric training. Whether you are new to exercise or an experienced bodybuilder, *Muscles in Minutes* will help you get bigger and stronger faster than you ever imagined. *Muscles in Minutes* is a complete fitness program for anyone who wants to build muscle.

Muscles in Minutes includes:
- Rapid-fire weight training exercises
- Accelerated cardiovascular training routines
- Time-saving meals that build muscle and burn fat
- Mental triggers that speed results
- Plus training programs that break through plateaus, and much, much more!

Negative training is a proven, tested way to gain explosive strength quickly and safely. Although the concept of forced negatives has been known to trainers and fitness specialists for years, *Muscles in Minutes* is the first book to utilize these powerful techniques to help men and women of all fitness levels achieve lasting results with minimal effort.

$15.95
ISBN 1-57826-137-6

MUSCLES IN MINUTES
The Insiders' Guide to Body Building with Negative Training
Steve Leamont

STEVE LEAMONT, a personal trainer with more than 15 years of experience, has trained with several bodybuilding champions. After years of studying, Steve pioneered the revolutionary technique presented now in *Muscles in Minutes*. He lives in Windsor, Ontario, Canada.

Available at bookstores everywhere

(if you don't see it, ask for it) or call toll-free:
1-800-906-1234

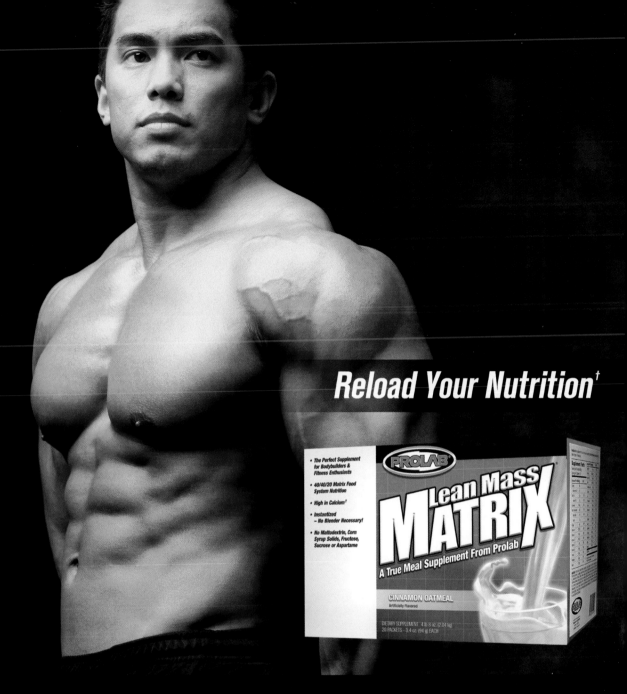

Reload Your Nutrition†

- *The Perfect Supplement for Bodybuilders & Fitness Enthusiasts*
- *40/40/20 Matrix Food System Nutrition*
- *High in Calcium*†
- *Instantized – No Blender Necessary!*
- *No Maltodextrin, Corn Syrup Solids, Fructose, Sucrose or Aspartame*

PROLAB

Lean Mass MATRIX

A True Meal Supplement From Prolab

CINNAMON OATMEAL
Artificially Flavored

DIETARY SUPPLEMENT 4 lb 8 oz. (2.04 kg)
20 PACKETS – 3.4 oz (94 g) EACH

Real results from a real meal supplement

...thanks to a perfect balance of protein, carbs and fats. This is no sugary, filler-laden, synthesized quickie drink – this is a true meal supplement, with macro nutrition that delivers the "definition of definition." Our **Lean Mass Matrix**® formula replenishes key vitamins and minerals while maintaining lean body mass.† And it delivers an ideal 40/40/20 ratio of protein, complex carbs and essential fats. Or try **Prolab**® **Naturally Lean Matrix**®, with the same balance of nutrition and about half the calories. Prolab has been building products like these that help you build the body you want since 1993.

Find out more. Join the VIP Club at www.prolab.com or call 1 800 PROLAB1

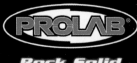

Rock Solid

† These statements have not been evaluated by the Food and Drug Administration. This product is not intended to diagnose, treat, cure or prevent any disease.

Try our great tasting Lean Mass Matrix® flavors for *FREE!*
Visit www.prolab.com/samples (while supplies last)

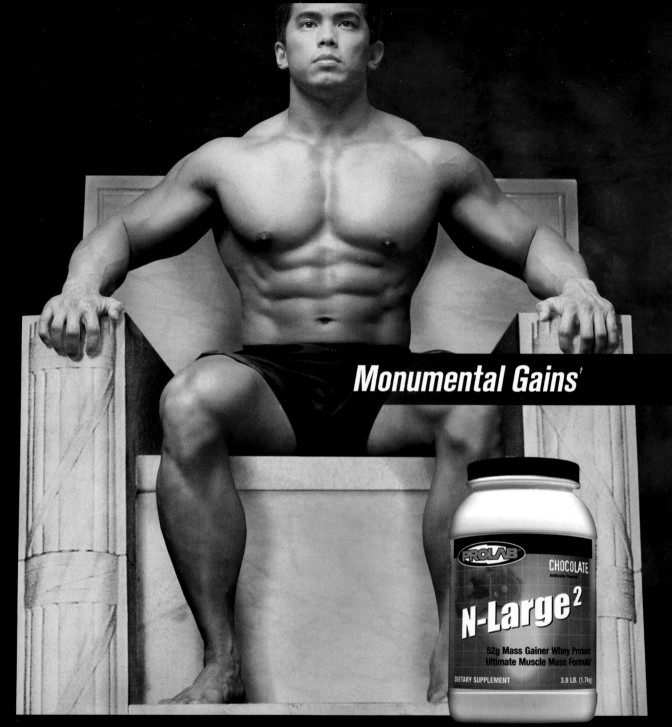

Monumental Gains[†]

You're bigger than life

Increasing lean muscle tissue comes from hard work and proper nutrition. You're ready for **Prolab®** **N-Large**[2], the mass-gaining support formula designed to help you gain weight and get big, not fat. Protein? Yeah, more than 50 grams per serving. It's the essential nutrient that promotes muscle mass. We've got the bioavailability you demand and whey protein with a superior amino acid profile, and mixing it up is a snap.[†] Prolab has been building products like these that help you build the body you want since 1993.

Find out more. Join the VIP Club at www.prolab.com or call 1 800 PROLAB1

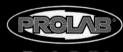

Rock Solid

[†] These statements have not been evaluated by the Food and Drug Administration. This product is not intended to diagnose, treat, cure or prevent any disease.

Try our *NEW* and improved N-Large[2] flavors for *FREE!*
Visit *www.prolab.com/samples* (while supplies last)